ABOUT THE AU

GAYE MACK, MA

Gaye has throughout her life had a deep interest in esoteric philosophies, spirituality in medicine, and healing, and was among the early group of practitioners in the United States to attain a place on the Dr Edward Bach Foundation International Register of Practitioners. She has a background of study in psychology and sociology. Gaye's Master of Arts degree in Integrated Professional Studies from DePaul University, Chicago, focused on holistic medicine with particular application of the Bach Remedies as an integrative therapy for eating disorders and other emotional illnesses.

She is the author of several articles published internationally on the Bach work, and is listed in Who's Who in Medicine and Healthcare, 2000, and Who's Who in America, 2003, 2004. In addition to her private practice, she regularly conducts workshops in North America and Great Britain.

Although she has travelled widely in Great Britain, Europe, India, Nepal, Africa and Egypt, she keeps her linen closet and her family in the Chicago, Illinois area.

Gaye may be contacted through:

Polair Publishing · P O Box 34886 · London W8 6YR

www.polairpublishing.co.uk

www.naturesbridge.com

naturesbridge@aol.com

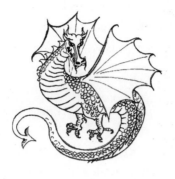

IGNITING SOUL FIRE

SPIRITUAL DIMENSIONS OF THE
BACH FLOWER REMEDIES

Gaye Mack, MA

Polair Publishing · London · England

First published May 2004 by Polair Publishing,
P O Box 34886, London W8 6YR
www.polairpublishing.co.uk

(c) Copyright, Nature's Bridge, Inc., 2004

British Library Cataloguing-in-Publication Data

A Catalogue record for this book is
available from the British Library

ISBN 0-9545389-2-7

Set in 12.5 on 16 pt Spectrum and printed in the UK
by Cambridge University Press

CONTENTS

Acknowledgments · vii

Preface · ix

Author's Note · xiii

ONE · Spiritual Law and Sacred Shopping · 15

TWO · Intuition is the Voice of the Soul · 24

THREE · From Medicine Man to Mystic · 37

FOUR · Here be Dragons · 52

FIVE · In the Name of Service and Brotherhood · 67

SIX · As Above, so Below · 77

SEVEN · The Seven Sacred Gates · 100

EIGHT · It's All in the Chakras · 109

NINE · Taking Root: the First Chakra · 115

TEN · Personal Best: the Second Chakra · 123

ELEVEN · Solar Power: the Third Chakra · 134

TWELVE · At the Crossroads: the Fourth Chakra · 146

THIRTEEN · Speak Loudly: the Fifth Chakra · 157

FOURTEEN · Light-bulb Moments: the Sixth Chakra · 165

FIFTEEN · Illumination: the Seventh Chakra · 175

SIXTEEN · Keep on Keeping on · 181

The 38 Bach Flower Remedies · 185

Practical Matters · 186

Selected Further Reading · 190

ACKNOWLEDGMENTS

These days, any new author finds it a most difficult challenge to create a work worthy of a publisher's attention. Actually to see it manifested into print is a gift. For this reason I am exceedingly grateful to Colum Hayward and Polair Publishing for providing the opportunity for *Igniting Soul Fire* to reach you. But before the print stage, the birthing process of every book needs a midwife and this one was no exception. *Igniting Soul Fire* would never have come to a reality were it not for my editor, Kärin Baltzell, supreme scholar, psychologist, intuitive, and exceptional *spirit*. Kärin manifests the true embodiment of 'doing service' on the front lines of the spiritual path and my gratitude to her for this 'service' is beyond measure. My added appreciation goes to Simon Bentley, Principal of the White Eagle School of Astrology in the UK, for his astrological expertise and insights regarding Edward Bach's natal chart. Fourthly, I am enormously grateful to Morgan Hesmondhalgh for the brilliance of her cover design and for the extraordinary ability in conjuring up dragons from nowhere and in no time!

As Edward Bach shows us, the practice of healing and medicine is a divinely-inspired art and gift. Should your path cross one who practises his/her craft with this understanding and in this spirit, you will be a very fortunate person, as I have been. For his care, his insights over the years and especially for introducing me to Edward Bach and his work, I am grateful to Jerry Gore, healer, physician, and very old soul. As it is said, there are no accidents.

I also owe a debt of gratitude to Professor Morry Fiddler of DePaul University, Chicago. During my graduate years, Morry was a constant support as I travelled through the scary waters of the unknowable, encouraging me to speak my truth in front of and in spite of, audiences filled with highly sceptical dragons. As a professor with a doctorate in genetics, Morry constantly badgered me by asking, 'How do you know'? To which I persistently replied, and still do, 'Because I just *know*'.

There are others of course who are deserving of my gratitude: many friends here in the US and 'across the pond', who have my appreciation for their blind encouragement and support while asking each other behind my back (Do you *get* what she is writing about?). At the risk of forgetting someone and specifically naming those who, for various reasons, I suspect wish to remain anonymous, I have made the decision to thank you as a collective. In any case, you all know who you are and I am deeply grateful.

And certainly last, but not the least in any way, I am so grateful for my husband and son who have put up with having to share their space with Edward Bach for all of these years. They deserve endurance medals, as they never bothered to whisper behind my back, but are quite up front in simply saying, 'yes, dear, yes, Mom ... uh huh'.

PREFACE

In the midst of my forties and what I thought was the 'dream' corporate job of my life, my health suddenly took a serious dive. As a result, I entered a period of several years during which I had numerous tests and was examined by many specialists. While each was well qualified in their field, none seemed to have the definitive answer and my health continued to deteriorate. Finally, a friend suggested that I seek out an evaluation by a local, western-trained physician who practised classical homeopathy and Ayurvedic medicine. This physician is the healer who is responsible for not only getting me on the path to whole health, but also introducing me to Edward Bach and his thirty-eight powerful flower remedies.

Attaining a state of balance in mind, body, and spirit requires an alchemical mix of tools in order to heal at each of these levels. My path was no exception. The exception for me, however, was that my initiation into Edward Bach's world and his work was the igniting of my own soul fire; and the rest, as they say, is history.

If Bach were physically with us today, I think he would be astonished at the global breadth his work has reached in the last seventy-plus years. Today there are several major flower-remedy repertoires around the globe. This does not count the thousands of individuals who prepare their own flower remedies from their gardens and the fields of nature, as Bach himself encouraged people to do. The fact that the discovery of flower-remedy therapy is universally acknowledged as exclusively his, speaks for the brilliance of Bach's work. Thus, with such expansion of his work have come many excellent resources to guide people throughout the world.

They are examining his discoveries, studying his guidelines, and using the formulas and remedies in their daily lives. Several of these resources are listed in 'Further Reading'.

Moreover, this book is not another manual to be placed along side these resources. Because of this, readers already familiar with Bach's thirty-eight remedies will notice that I have not included examination of the Seven Helpers, nor have I included all of the Final Nineteen remedies as application examples. I have, however, provided a brief section on the practical details of Bach therapy so that you may easily add it to your personal resources on healing.

I feel an explanation regarding the visual style and some of the metaphorical images used within the text, might be useful. As *Igniting* took shape, it became clear that the cover would have to convey the message that this is not the usual book on flower remedies with beautiful flowers on the front. As a result, the cover was intended to reflect the ultimate healing message of the Star of Bethlehem as a remedy for all of us as we enter the Age of Aquarius, the flower's mystical image of a six-pointed star of balance and the phoenix of our soul fire rising into the heavens. And then came the dragons.

As I wrote *Igniting*, many things just presented themselves. Using dragons as a symbolic metaphor for our difficult emotions throughout was one of them. It was not until I began the proofreading phase that I realized Bach himself referred to the 'dragon of fear', something I quote in the Author's Notes; a section written after the main text was finished. As a result, the editorial decision was made to include dragons a primary visual imagery. As visuals, if nothing else, they are there constantly to remind us of our necessary work as we travel on our mystical journey.

Finally, a few remarks on syntax used in the pages that follow are necessary. In Bach's day, attention to being politically correct regarding gender specifics in writing and speaking simply did not happen. Today, of course, there is a great deal of attention paid to such details. In order to enhance the flow of thought, I have not attempted to insert notations such as he/she in Bach's quotes or references to them. I felt this would be extremely cumbersome and detract from the more important concepts. Thus, it should be understood by the reader that any reference to 'he' is meant to include the feminine as well. This perspective also applies to the term, 'brotherhood'. Clearly, as the Aquarian Age approaches, more than ever, this term includes the universality of all of us in human form, regardless of gender.

There is little doubt that Bach's gift as a healer and his discovery of the remedies were divinely originated. Daily life on this planet has changed tremendously for most of us since Bach's death and there are many who have expanded his original thirty-eight remedies into larger systems. It is common, as a practitioner, to hear remarks suggesting that Bach's work is out of date or out of touch with the times. This rationale suggests that we live in a world-climate far different from Edward Bach's and that, as a result, we have many more challenges emotionally. Some suggest that our energetic vibrations are shifting at a faster rate than Bach could have imagined. While I do not dispute that we are indeed living in very different times, we are still human, and the emotions of the human condition have not evolved into something new. Rather, we now find that difficult emotions occur with more frequency and at a higher level of intensity.

The circumstances creating such experiences are complex. We live in a world where our ecology, our security, and our health are under constant threat. While many in the world suffer from hunger, the rest of us who are well fed are at risk nutritionally owing to the damaging ways our food supply is manipulated. Thus, in addition to the emotional stresses of our external environment, many of us lack proper nutrition, which results in the body chemistry creating emotional roller-coaster rides. Despite the passage of time, the range of our emotions is the same today as it was in Dr Bach's era: we are at times terrified, become depressed or angry; we exhibit rage, and we experience detachment, joy, grief, and loneliness.

Bach was a healer who recognized that divinity or a divine spark exists in each of us. His intent was to make us aware of this divinity and to teach us further about the gentle divinity of nature and its ability to heal. His beliefs are steeped in simplicity, for in simplicity we find truth. Living in the age of speed and technology, we sometimes forget that we create a picture so complex that the simple solutions evade us.

Furthermore, the intent of this book is not to debate the value of those who have followed in Bach's footsteps. In fact, Bach knew that others would come after him in their attempts to 'improve' upon his work:

> *As soon as a teacher has given his work to the world, a contorted version of the same must arise. . . . [This version] must be raised for people to be able to choose between the gold and the dross.*

Instead, the pages that follow explore the relationship between the deeper aspects of the remedies and their ability to help us find 'the high truth of our soul fire'. This work delves deeply into Bach's own nature as a mystic and the gifts as a healer that were so much a part of him.

With the Age of Aquarius and its energy upon us, many of us find that we are compelled to explore our own spirituality and soul-purpose for this lifetime. The questions before us are how can we heal our karmic debts and, at the same time, discover our own divinity in the quest for universal brotherhood/sisterhood.

Bach was very clear and determined in following his own soul-path despite the difficulties it posed. I hope that the pages before you will encourage you to open your heart to your own healing and, at the very least, kindle the flames of inspiration that are waiting in your own soul. In this effort, I have endeavoured to show how deeply spiritual and introspective Bach's thoughts and writings were. In addition, you will find presented the valuable guidelines he offers us as we seek healing and progress in our own spiritual growth. It is important to remember that each moment of breath is an opportunity. What we choose in that moment is that which determines our next step.

I hope he is pleased.

GFM
March 2004

AUTHOR'S NOTES

Two of the questions I often hear from my clients and those who attend my workshops are, if Bach was such a great healer, what did he die from and why did he die so young? From a physical standpoint Bach's health was always an issue and as discussed in this book, his death certificate notes cardiac failure and sarcoma. However, from a spiritual perspective, mystics and visionaries often 'sense' that the time for their earthly work is drawing to a close and do not fear their transition. Certainly, no less was true of Edward Bach.

Shortly before his death, Bach wrote several letters to friends, colleagues and business associates that seem to imply that he was 'tidying up things' in preparation for his transition. Certainly, since he was a physician, it is not unreasonable to assume that he was well aware of his physical status. But in the letters that follow, one gets the sense that he was in a place that was far outside the density of the physical realm:

> *I am expecting a call to a work more congenial than of this very difficult world.... The Work I have put before you is Great Work, it God's Work, and heaven only knows why I should be called away at this moment to continue to fight for suffering humanity.* *

*Original writings, p. 173.

And this; written only one month to the day before his passing.

October 26, 1936

Dear Folk,

It would be wonderful to form a little Brotherhood without rank or office, none greater and none less than the other, who devoted themselves to the following principles:

1. That there has been disclosed unto us a System of Healing such as has not been known within the memory of men; when, with the simplicity of the Herbal Remedies, we can set forth with the certainty, the absolute certainty, of their power to conquer disease.

2. That we never criticise nor condemn the thoughts, the opinions, the ideas of others; ever remembering that all humanity are God's children, each striving in his own way to find the Glory of his Father. That we set out on the one hand, as knights of old, to destroy the dragon of fear, knowing that we may never have one discouraging word, but that we can bring hope, aye and most of all, certainty to those who suffer.

3. That we never get carried away by praise or success that we meet in our Mission, knowing that we are but the messengers of the Great Power.

4. That as more and more we gain the confidence of those around, we proclaim to them we believe that we are divine agents sent to succour them in their need.

5. That as people become well, that the Herbs of the field which are healing them, are the gift of Nature which is the Gift of God; thus bring them back to a belief in the love, the mercy, and the tender compassion and the almighty power of the most high.

EDWARD BACH*

*Barnard, *Collected Writings*, p. 170.

CHAPTER ONE

SPIRITUAL LAW
AND SACRED SHOPPING

*We are a culture of spiritual seekers, closet mystics and sacred
shoppers. But, you say, this culture has been around for eons. Well, yes;
but not like we see it today. The Age of Aquarius is approaching,
bringing with it energy that compels us to shift our personal energy to
one that lives the consciousness of universal brotherhood. Shift of
consciousness is the real news. This consciousness, for each of us, is a
journey of our emotions, of our Sacred Contract, forged between soul
and spirit, for the emotions are the gateway to the spiritual.*

IN ANCIENT astrology individual spirit, the timeless Divine
Spark encased in matter of the human body, was symbol-
ized as a dot within a circle. This symbol is still used by modern astrologers. Additionally, esoteric teachings tell us that
our spirit has engaged in a contract with our soul and that a
principle of this contract commands that we follow a path
keenly orchestrated within a framework of five cosmic laws,
that of *Rebirth, Karma, Opportunities, Balance and Correspondence.* And
it is on this journey that our soul, our spiritual heart, holds
continuous precise records of our experiences and lessons.
These records are available for us to draw upon as a resource.
If we use this resource, we have opportunities to develop

depth to our wisdom and are able to move forward in our growth. The law of *Rebirth* determines that each of us remain in the natural cycle of birth, death and earthly rebirth until that time when we attain a state of final transcendence beyond this cycle. This transcendence can only occur when we have completed our path of soul-awareness and discovery of our personal High Truth and soul-purpose.

So what is the catch? The catch is that it is through the body that we are compelled to learn our necessary soul-lessons, for in order to discover our High Truth and soul-purpose we must *feel*. In order to transcend and stop repeating the human life cycle we need to be in the body so that we can experience all ranges of emotions and, thus, feel.

Spiritual teachings state that the soul is the feminine aspect of the self. It is through this aspect that the Divine intends us to connect with our emotional self. During each lifetime, the experience of our physical body brings us the extremes of joy and pain. It is through these emotional experiences that each one of us has the opportunity to access the feminine aspect of the self. Further, the range of emotions available to us brings value to our soul-growth and self-empowerment.

Emotions are what develop our intuition, sometimes referred to as our 'sixth sense'. In the Age of Aquarius and the energy that will accompany it, intuition will be the path of communication and understanding. While some inspirational writers and teachers imply that we are already in this Age, the reality is that we are not quite there yet. If we step back so that we have a global view, it is not difficult to see that our attitudes of the past and in the present not only affect our lives and the lives of others, but they have a direct correlation to the embryonic level of our awareness and sensitivity to this soul-resource of intuition.

Within each lifetime, each one of us consciously and unconsciously experiences our emotional landscape externally and internally. These landscapes are in constant motion, interactive, and profoundly affect how we function in the mundane world. More importantly, these emotional landscapes become a reflection of our relationship to the five Cosmic Laws that challenge us to consider the consequences of not connecting to our emotional self.

The Law of *Karma* purposely places us in circumstances and relationships within each incarnation whereby we sow and reap future consequences of emotional and physical interaction with others we have wronged or abused. Equally, we find that within each incarnation we again meet those whom we have loved or who have loved us. These are the encounters that bring us joy. It is important for us, however, to recognize that past wrongs cannot be rectified, or joy in relationships appreciated, if we are not able consciously to come to terms with our own emotions. Therefore, it is through these experiences and relationships that our soul propels us toward the awareness of what it means to *feel*.

Every situation or interaction with others requires a decision as to whether each of us will respond with malice or kindness, hate or love. Consciously or unconsciously, our emotional self drives these decisions. We can think of this particular law functioning like a set of karmic scales. How we respond to our internal and external environment through thought and action affects the balance of these scales and thus, the direction of our future path.

In its divine wisdom, our soul readily provides us circumstances in which we are presented not only with opportunities to pay off karmic debt incurred by past transgressions but we are also able to balance out our karmic debts positively through love and kindness. This is the *law of opportunity* and we are given freewill within the boundaries of this law. But surprisingly, during our human experience, we come up against unexpected detours from the way we envisaged things would work out for us during this experience. We find that while we bask in the light of some achievements, more often than not the journey is one that is fraught with disappointments and shattered dreams from unrealized expectations. This simply is because they are not part of our soul's plan for us this lifetime. Two keys to our soul-growth are found in both our reactions and actions to circumstances and life events. In other words, *our responses in thought and action have an effect on the balance of our karmic scale.*

From a spiritual perspective, our soul is concerned with the concept of balance and so it is that we are placed from lifetime to lifetime in environments that can vastly differ, swinging from one end of the spectrum to the other. For example, in one lifetime an individual may find that life is easy and wealth accessible, and in the next they may be homeless. These lifetimes however, composed of vastly-opposing elements, support us in the process of recognizing our emotional responses to life-events, in addition to the effect of our actions toward others. It is in this awareness as these lifetimes play out that we build up the resource of wisdom. This is the *law of balance.*

We now come to the fifth law, that of *Correspondences.* It is this law which summarizes the basic principles of the other four. Healing is the balance of mind, body and spirit for others and for oneself through unconditional love. But working toward this state, even if we are aware of the goal, is not easy. In its divine wisdom, our soul constantly sends us messages through these five cosmic laws within each lifetime. The problem is that when we do not get the message or see the opportunities we can become frustrated, angry, or fearful with what appears to be roadblocks that surround us.

Driven to find answers in the midst of our frustration, soul-pressure, malcontent and other feelings, we become seekers, closet mystics, and *sacred shoppers.* We read, we practice postures, we meditate, and pray. We study the stars and are inspired by psychics, rituals and stones. We follow gurus and diets. We join circles and ashrams, never finding answers that seem to resonate with us; because in our frenetic search for the one thing that will ignite our soul's fire, our emotions become just as frenetic as our search. In our quest, we recall that some reference to exploring our emotional self has been made, but the idea of this excavation is put on the back burner. It seems too scary or we may not like what we find. There are dragons down there. So in our anxiety we revert to where it is safe; the place where we believe we can maintain control of ourselves and everything around us: the mind.

When I lecture on the subject of discovering soul fire, I often use the metaphorical image of embarking on a spiritual journey that requires 'boarding the spiritual train.' Exploring one's spiritual self creates anxiety for many, and in this anxiety we are so afraid that the spiritual train will leave without us that we never hear our soul whisper the key:

balance between our mind and emotions is the path to our high truth, our wisdom, and our soul-purpose. It is not an issue of heart versus mind. It is an issue of working in harmony, of learning to listen with the heart and *then* acting with the mind.

The divine universe works on a 'need to know' basis that is not in the business of giving us access to the whole picture. The lack of access to such trajectory vision *is* the divine plan for each of us, honed to perfection by a Divinity that never misses opportunities to humble us just when we think that we know it all. In Native American mythology this cosmic posture is embodied in the Coyote, otherwise identified as the 'trickster'. This rascal tricks us into believing we know the scheme and then playfully pulls the cosmic rug right out from under us. However, we do have recourse, and it is this: while no spiritual train will leave without us, we have to be willing to leave the platform of the station and in faith, in the unconscious and improvable knowing, climb on board with our karmic baggage.

On our journey, we have to be willing to explore the emotions this journey reveals to us—the unhealed conflicts within us—and be willing to participate in the transformation of our toxic patterns so that we can embrace our High Truth. This is what soul-path is about. This is living on purpose. But living on purpose and the process of emotional discovery is a challenge in itself; and often we are not equipped to work alone. Being receptive to accepting assistance from those who can interpret, witness, and guide us is invaluable. Help of this sort that is worth considering may lie in various forms of therapy, including bodywork, art therapy, psychotherapy, or consulting a spiritual advisor.

In addition to these options that are certainly not exclusive ones, our resources should also include Dr Bach's Flower remedies. It is these 'God-sent Gift(s)' as Bach described them* that offer us a 'safety-net' as we explore our emotional self. Consideration of the remedies is important because once we have made the decision to explore our spiritual self, our journey can be a ride of emotional extremes. We find that our landscape varies between peacefulness and times of roaring through dark tunnels. In this darkness, we cannot see; and it is in these moments that we want to jump off the train, thinking we'll take another one or do 'it' another time. The difficulty is that once we have committed to this journey our Contract ensures that we must be present; we must participate in the process and there is no going back or getting off. Our experiences however, are only the wrapping paper that encloses the gift of heart wisdom. The Universe is clever, in that in order to access the wisdom that is held within the soul, our spiritual heart, we have to remove the outer wrappings. This process—and it is a process—is the alchemy of our journey.

As we travel our path, our soul continues to whisper messages to us, but we find it difficult if not impossible to hear them, as we have a hard time surrendering our Mental Plan to our soul's plan. As we continue in our resistance, our external environment becomes difficult, forewarning us that we must shift our emotional perspective. Somehow we don't get the message, ignoring the warnings to shift our perspective. Finally, unheeded, these soul-messages begin to manifest in difficult life-events and/or relationships. Our emotions

* *The Twelve Healers,* p. 3 .

begin to reel unpleasantly out of balance, and then it is only a matter of time before the body ceases to function in a balanced way. The medical intuitive, Carolyn Myss, Ph.D., has a wonderful expression that personifies this principle: 'your biography is your biology'. In other words, if we don't excavate our emotional distress and our karmic baggage, our body will reflect our resistance. For some of us, this means experiencing longer illnesses in order to learn necessary lessons for our soul-growth. For others of us, the framework of these needed lessons may come in a combination of both external material and internal physical difficulties.

Another way of expressing this principle is to remember that whatever is happening to us internally will be mirrored in our external environment; the microcosm is a reflection of the macrocosm. *This is the Law of Correspondences.*

In those moments when we are brought to a state of crisis, whether it is emotional, physical, or both, we are brought to the edge of our personal abyss. *The Tibetan Book of Living and Dying* by Sogyal Rinpoche reminds us that to follow the path of our wisdom has never been more difficult; we do not live in a world that supports this. We live in a world that seems to be anchored in the mind, rather than the heart, and yet operating from the spiritual heart has never before been so imperative.*The Aquarian energy that we are coming into compels each of us to jump into our personal abyss, taking the leap of faith as individuals and as the collective human race.

As we teeter on the edge of our abyss, not just once, but repeatedly; as we ignore our soul-messages, our fear and despair reflect beliefs that we don't have operating instructions, maps or tools to manage the next right step. These beliefs, fuelled by the Trickster, the crazy-maker, create havoc anchored in our emotional body. In our fears and terrors the ego tells us that we are headed for disaster if we take the risk of embracing a leap of faith. Nevertheless, the ego fighting for control does not recognize that we are in divine protective custody and in this custody, we have instructions, tools, and maps; we just have to learn how to recognize the instructions found in the wisdom of our spiritual heart.

Established in the yogic tradition, the concept of chakras is now widely accepted across most spiritual philosophies and by some practitioners of western medicine. These seven major centres of energy (and hundreds of minor ones) are actually mirrors of our emotional patterns that are reflected in a condition of expansion or contraction. Whether the emotional essence of a chakra is balanced (expanded) or unbalanced (contracted) has a direct effect upon our physical state of wellness (or not). The Bach remedies are powerful tools that assist us to bring about a balance in the chakras, and they increase in us an awareness of soul-messages through chakra-patterns. In other words, they ignite the soul's fire.

As we gain clarity in understanding the relationship between the emotional maps mirrored in our chakras and the balancing effect of the remedies, we can begin to engage in the process of bringing our body, mind, and spirit into harmony. The architecture of this process in discovering our soul's fire and high truth was *known* and well understood by Edward Bach, physician, healer ... *mystic.*

CHAPTER TWO

INTUITION IS THE VOICE
OF THE SOUL

THERE IS A Buddhist expression from the fifth or sixth century that goes like this: 'All know the way, few actually walk it' (Bodhidharma). Listening to our intuition, our 'soul's voice,' is part of walking the 'way'. Unfortunately, traditional society has only supported this concept by weak acknowledgment that listening to our intuition is a philosophy best left to the religious and business communities. At worst, traditionalists believe it is a malady of self-professed psychics and nutcases. For those of us who are not self-professed psychics and don't believe we are nutcases, learning to listen to our intuition is not only a tricky business; it can be a risky business. Nevertheless, each of us has a soul-job and none of us is here by accident, although sometimes we believe that we are. Whatever the soul-agenda, it centres on transmuting karmic debt, taking it in, taking it on, inhaling it, and incorporating it into our soul-growth. This takes us to a deeper, higher level of understanding, bringing us closer to home on our journey; recalling that, indeed, we are spirit.

There are days when we can feel that the totality of our soul-mission is the job of self-healing, for the pain is so deep that there is no room or energy for anyone or anything else.

It is days like this when we forget, if indeed we have ever learned, how to listen to our soul's voice, our intuition. This voice is here to guide us, particularly in times of extreme life-challenges and lessons. It is also easy to assume that those who truly walk their intended soul-path do so with some sort of special dispensation. This is simply not the case. We can look to Edward Bach as someone who not only knew the way, but also walked it despite disappointments, rejection, and obstacles. Edward Bach was one who quite clearly functioned within the framework of the five cosmic laws. In other words, like the rest of us, he had no special dispensation. In fact, it was quite the opposite. Bach held the fierce belief that intuition is the voice of our soul. Not only did he *know* this philosophy, but also he unquestionably lived it. A great deal of current research informs us that intent on the part of the healer plays an important role in the effectiveness of the therapy and influence upon the intended individual. While we may feel bombarded with a plethora of choices in our sacred shopping, finding a truly gifted healer is not easy.

What is a 'gifted healer?' Gifted healers use their intuition, natural skills, and knowledge with selfless intent and purpose to assist others in the discovery of their *high truth* and soul's fire through a balanced connection between their emotional mind and their intuitive heart. Certainly there is no doubt that Edward Bach was an extraordinarily-gifted healer who passionately believed that intuition and the voice of our soul are one and the same.*

Further, it is important for us to understand that Bach's

*Original Writings, p. 44.

spiritual beliefs and soul-path are reflected in the discovery of the remedies. Keeping in mind that the mission of our soul-path is to teach us how to feel, is it any wonder that the Bach Remedies are about this very thing; teaching us to participate, reflect upon and embrace our emotions through opportunities that invite us to transform toxic patterns from our past? In addition, in this process we just may discover our soul's fire and intended path for this life.

A great many books are available that inform us about Edward Bach's career as an orthodox physician and the course of events leading to his groundbreaking discovery of the Remedies between 1928 and 1935. Unfortunately, material is scant that extensively details his interest in matters of the esoteric or his explicit personal and spiritual connection to the plants and their resulting remedies. This lack of information may be due in part, as Julian Barnard points out, to the fact that Bach was most probably a very private individual in such matters. * But, in spite of this deficiency, we can glean some insights about him. Though lacking in specific details, Bach's two small books, *Heal Thyself,* and *The Twelve Healers* (which relate exclusively to the remedies), express his spiritual philosophy within a broader framework.

Additionally, the author Nora Weeks, who worked closely with Bach during the remedy years (1928–1935), wrote two books about him and his work. Although she clearly preserves an untarnished portrait of the man whom she so obviously respected professionally and personally, there is a lack of enlightenment over some personal details. There is no mention of any personal relationships Bach had, other

*Barnard, 2002.

than professional ones. Weeks indicates that Bach was a committed Freemason, believed in past lives, astrology, and other esoteric subjects, yet more details that are expansive simply are not forthcoming from her. In all fairness, however, it is likely that we might have even less knowledge about Bach if it were not for Nora Weeks. Following his death in the autumn of 1936, along with the small group of supporters who had worked with Bach and the remedies over the years, Nora Weeks carried on the work at Mount Vernon (today known as the Dr Bach Centre) in accordance with Bach's request.

As a young radiographer, Weeks left London with Bach in 1930 as his assistant when he made the decision to abandon orthodox medicine in pursuit of discovering a simple and pure system of healing. In her book, *The Medical Discoveries of Edward Bach, Physician,* Weeks relates details of Bach's story as a physician and his discovery of the Remedies.

From the time he was young, Bach *knew* that his path was that of a healer; it was just a question of whether he would seek this path through medicine or the church. Fortunately for us, he chose medicine, obtaining the combined diplomas of M.R.C.S. and L.R.C.P. in 1912 followed by the degrees of M.B., B.S. (1913) and Ph. D. (Cambridge, 1913). During his years in London as a medical man, his reputation grew so much that he was allocating his time between his consulting practice on Harley Street and his research laboratory at Park Crescent. By 1928, Edward Bach had come to a point in his professional career where he had been recognized and honoured, both in the UK and abroad, with distinction for his work in bacteriology, immunology, pathology, and finally homeopathy.

However, there was another side to Bach, and it is here the story becomes intriguing. Even as a very young man, Bach was a keen observer of human nature, and he seemed to possess a highly-developed intuitive sense about the suppressed emotional states of those around him. In his later years as a physician, this 'sense' extended to an awareness of obscured physical imbalances in others. Today, he surely would be regarded as a medical intuitive and probably a psychic as well. While his success as an orthodox physician and man of science grew in traditional circles, a major shift occurred in his experience with medicine in the later 1920s that had a tremendous impact on the direction his life was to take.

Weeks relates that at this point he had become increasingly dissatisfied with the methods utilized by those that practised traditional medicine. Privately, as a student of the esoteric, healing for him had become something other than a matter of treating the symptomology of illness or disease. For Bach, it was a matter of treating soul and spirit as well. In observing his patients, he had come to recognize that there was a definite connection between the emotional state of his patients and their chronic illnesses.

These observations led him to formulate his theory on the origins of illness and disease in the light of his belief that they were a result of disharmony between the soul and the personality. Further, he was adamant that the method of regaining wellness came through harmonizing this disharmony. In fact, integrating the soul and the personality was the key to avoiding illness altogether. He was also convinced that nature held the keys to attaining this harmony. It was as if, in addition to what knowledge he had of the esoteric, he *intuitively knew* that the soul's message is to teach us how to feel. Through this process of both painful and joyful emotions, we develop our intuitive sixth sense, the voice of our soul. It would appear that this conscious awareness of the relationship between the soul and the personality was an indication of his own expanding awareness and the soul-path intended for him.

If we consider what we know of Bach's personal history within the context of the Five Cosmic Laws, it is possible to get a glimpse of the path intended for him by his soul. This consideration is important. Bearing in mind that the intent of the healer has a direct impact upon the healing process and its outcome, consideration of Bach's intent and spiritual orientation is valuable in understanding the simple but profound healing potential provided by the remedies. Interestingly, just as it is useful for us to consider the framework of Bach and his work from a different perspective, the core message of his remedies is about shifting our emotional perception or framework in order to pursue the discovery of our own soul-path.

Furthermore, if we reflect on some of Bach's personality characteristics, we can additionally begin to see how the *laws of rebirth, karma, opportunity, balances and correspondences* played out in his life. For example, as a young man, Bach had a very difficult time within the city environment. His state of health was always an issue, manifesting from minor to extreme life-threatening circumstances throughout his life until his death at the early age of fifty. Nora Weeks' accounts of Bach's personality relate his intense dislike of the city environment,

and his constant struggle with a central nervous system that
was very fragile and, moreover, one that was only soothed
by the natural environment. Fragile nervous systems are
not unusual in individuals who are gifted with the heightened intuitive nature found in psychics, but also those
who have the gift of clairvoyance or ability to see images or
visions.

We know from material available that he suffered chronic
physical ailments in the early years of his medical career,
and particularly during the years he worked exclusively with
the remedies (1928–1935). She reports him as saying to her,
'Are you ever unconscious of your body?' When she replied,
'Yes', he continued by saying, 'You do not know how fortunate you are. All my life my body has suffered in some way
from pain and discomfort and distress.... I must know what
pain is like and experience every kind to have a true understanding of what others suffer.'*

After the initial discovery of the first nineteen remedies
in the repertoire, from 1928 to 1933, Bach then went on to
discover the final nineteen in 1934 and 1935. This latter period was extremely difficult for him both emotionally and
physically. Prior to the discovery of a new remedy during
this time, he would experience episodes that were debilitating physically and emotionally, according to Weeks:

> For many days during the hottest period of the summer his body was com-
> pletely covered by a virulent rash which burned and irritated incessantly; and
> for some weeks his legs were ulcerated, raw from knee to ankle; his hair came
> out and his sight almost failed. Before the finding of another remedy, his face
> was swollen and extremely painful. A severe haemorrhage exhausted him and

*Original Writings, p. 180-81

the bleeding did not cease until the remedy for the mental state he was passing through was found. *

In spite of the precarious nature of his health, professionally and personally, Bach was a man whom we would describe today as a workaholic. This pattern was one that was not only evident during his years of medical study, but also stayed with him until he announced in 1935 that his work with the remedies was complete. While this behaviour severely taxed the state of his health, this pattern and cost most likely were inevitable from a soul-path perspective. Interestingly, but not surprisingly, we find these similar patterns and constitutions in gifted healers within all cultures and traditions.

Bach, however, did find relief for mind, body and soul in the freedom he found in the countryside. To him, nature was Divine. He believed his highly-developed intuitive sense in working with patients and the healing qualities and vibrations of the remedies were a Divine gift of nature. His words reflect his humility, for he never referred to the remedies or their discovery as uniquely his. Rather he viewed himself simply as a channel or conduit for:

those Herbs of the field placed for Healing, by comforting, by soothing, by relieving our cares, our anxieties, [bringing] us nearer to the Divinity within. And it is that increase of the Divinity within which heals us ... thus we can truly say that certain Herbs have been placed for us by Divine Means, and the help which they give to us, not only heals our bodies, but brings into our lives, our characters, attributes of our Divinity. †

We can see the laws of *rebirth* and *karma* at work in Bach's

*Weeks, *Medical Discoveries*, p. 116. †Masonic Lecture, 1936, in Barnard, *Collected Writings*, p 13.

recollection of past incarnations. In these recollections, he said he had always been a healer, although Nora Weeks notes that these memories meant little to him. Seemingly, he was more concerned with the work he had come back to accomplish, because his work with the remedies could be passed onto others. However, his particular gifts of healing and 'sight', which he also acknowledged, were, as he put it, 'in higher hands' and could not be passed on to others.* Considering that he spent numerous past lives as a healer, we can surmise that his karmic mission in this life involved the task of providing all human beings with tools for their own self-healing. We know from esoteric writings that humanity through the ages has been given healing tools that far exceed our current knowledge and application. However, because of power struggles and abuse, they have 'gone underground' until such time when they could be rediscovered and used honourably.

While Nora Weeks reports that Bach was a Freemason, she does not detail his esoteric interests much beyond mentioning his affection for his Masonic brothers and his recollection of past lives as a healer. Julian Barnard however tells that Bach's esoteric interests covered a far larger sphere. Bach had quite an interest in astrology and originally felt that the distinctiveness of each of the Twelve Great Healers (the first twelve remedies) was unique because of the influence of the twelve signs of the zodiac.† In addition to his interest in astrology, he apparently embraced teachings of the Lord Buddha, Christ, and the Great Masters.§

---

*Original Writings pp. 181–2. †Barnard, Collected Writings, pp. 77–78. §Barnard, 2002, p. 29.

Clearly, Bach worked and wrote within a metaphysical framework. Further evidence of this is unmistakable in his reference to the collective of evolved souls known in metaphysical spirituality as the 'White Brotherhood'. In a letter written to a 'Brother' (presumably a fellow Mason) in 1934, Bach describes his anxiety for the future and that while lying 'near the tow-path at Marlow-on-Thames' a 'message came through'. He goes on to explain that this message was not only for himself, but also for all of those 'who are striving to help'. It is at this moment that he comprehends the brilliance of a gorse bush that is within his sight. He adds to his comments that the Gorse remedy was the first of the Four Helpers. *(Bach's Gorse remedy is recommended for hopelessness).* Bach concludes his letter by stating that this experience would mean nothing to many people, but to him it was a clear indication of how 'the White Brotherhood work, amongst us, not by miracles, not by apparitions, but by just leading us, if we are willing to be led, by every-day affairs'.* While Bach's personal philosophy was governed by such metaphysical depths, Barnard accurately states that, 'not everyone will continue with him on the journey'.† Nevertheless, his remedies are powerful regardless of one's personal philosophy.

Bach's break with orthodox medicine is not only evidence of his belief in the significance of listening to one's intuition, but additionally, it was the very embodiment of the *law of opportunity*. With his interest in the wider scope of esoteric philosophy, there can be little doubt that Bach saw his departure from orthodox medicine as an opportunity to pay off

*Original Writings, p. 92. †Barnard, 2002, p. 78.

old karmic debts. Further, of great importance, is that it gave
him the opportunity to see the larger picture of healing
humanity through nature. He was aware as well that opportunity did not mean a 'free ride'. He viewed opportunities from the spiritual perspective, in that they often appear
to us cloaked in difficulties and obstacles. However, they are
always for good reason:

> *Interferences occur in every life, they are part of the Divine Plan: they are
> necessary so that we can learn to stand up to them: in fact, we can look upon
> them as really useful opponents, merely there to help us gain in strength and
> realize our Divinity and our invincibility . . . the more apparent difficulties in
> our path we may be certain that our mission is worthwhile.* *

If we recall that Bach based the keystone of his theory of
illness and disease upon the concept of conflicts between
the soul and personality (or mind), we can see that Bach
virtually brings to our attention the essence of the *law of balance* in his remedies and likewise, the consequence of imbalance. His guide for healing was found in the balance of
nature. In one account, Weeks refers to Bach being 'shown'
the remedies. She cites that on one particular occasion, he
apparently was in a mood that was withdrawn and aloof,
when he suddenly announced that they would go in search
of the flower to help this state. Upon finding 'water violet'
Bach simply placed his hand over the flower and 'felt' what
we might understand as a symbiotic resonance bringing him
'a sense of peace, calmness, and humility.'†

Barnard refers to these occasions as inner teachings, but
regardless of the language, it is clear that Bach had a rapport with nature that was in concert with his soul-path.*

*Original Writings, p. 45: 'Free Thyself'. †Barnard, 2002, p 36–37.

He recognized that the life-force of certain flowers had the ability to balance out specific distressful and toxic emotions, so that we may 'never know disease or illness'. If we step back a moment and consider Bach's intent through his work, we can see that he was a man who constantly sought a state of balance in all things and believed that the key to finding balance was listening to our intuition.

Sadly, it seems, we find the *law of correspondences* mirrored in his lifelong struggle with his health. It is ironic that despite his genius and extraordinary gift as a healer, his own health was his greatest nemesis. This law reflects Bach's entire theory of illness and disease in that if we cannot reconcile internal toxic emotions, and repair the disconnection between mind and soul, the body will eventually reflect this and break down. 'We each have a Divine mission in this world, and our souls use our minds and bodies as instruments to do this work, so that when all three are working in unison the result is perfect health and perfect happiness.'†

It is difficult to grasp why good health eluded him. It is even harder to believe that listed on his death certificate as the causes of his demise were sarcoma (cancer) and cardiac arrest.§ Louise Hay, in You *Can Heal Your Life,* ascribes cancer to deep unresolved pain and grief, carrying deep hurts. Carolyn Myss, in *Anatomy of the Spirit,* cites numerous physical imbalances as they relate to the chakras and their emotional patterns. We can only surmise that in this lifetime Edward Bach was somehow repaying enormous karmic debt on many levels. It is unfortunate that his profession, which at one time had so honoured and respected him, abandoned

*Barnard, 2002., p. 36. †Original Writings, p. 41. §Barnard, 2002, p. 307.

him in the end when he began to speak his truth. Even more ironic is that today, he surely would be respected as a brilliant mind/body physician in the field of psychonueroimmunology.

Bach was a man who did not view life through a tunnel but envisioned the entire universe. Whatever he learned, it seems that it was never enough. He concluded in 1935 that for this lifetime his work was finished. Bach *knew* that his time in this incarnation was coming to a close in the fall of 1936. He wrote of this to a friend that he was expecting 'a call to a work more congenial than of this very difficult world'.* His gift to us is this beautiful system of healing and the teachings that encourage us to listen to our soul through our intuition. In all of his humility, his burning desire was to leave all human beings with a way to heal themselves. It is doubtful that he ever saw himself as the mystic that he was.

*Original Writings, p. 173.

CHAPTER THREE

FROM MEDICINE MAN TO MYSTIC

As we review our sacred shopping list searching for *the one practice or philosophy* that will spark or ignite our soul's fire, we find our list is bombarded with a plethora of shamans, psychics, channels for sentient beings from the other side, clairvoyants, clairaudients, seers, and—yes—mystics. While some are sincere pilgrims, sadly, others are ill-advised charlatans who perhaps will find their way in the next incarnation. Thus, on our quest, discrimination is an important tool to have at hand, with the bottom line being, *how do we know? What qualifies one as a mystic?* Moreover, how do we know that Edward Bach was one? What exactly are the prerequisites for mystic status? Are only saints qualified for this lofty-sounding mantle, or is one a mystic first then a saint? Well certainly, mysticism and sainthood are connected. But, if someone is not a saint, does this eliminate them from candidacy as a mystic? Or, if one is a saint, are they automatically a mystic? Certainly, this issue can easily become confusing.

Well, then, lots of suffering and solitude must be prerequisites (these are good ones). Yes, but not always. Portraying an individual as a mystic (and in some cases, believing oneself is a mystic) is all too familiar these days. Therefore, because of this rush to reverence, definition of mystical characteristics is significant. This detection is important in order that we may learn why Bach was a mystic. More importantly, how did this state of consciousness affect him as he worked with the remedies; and how in turn, do they have an effect on us?

In 1911, Evelyn Underhill wrote her classic, *Mysticism, the Nature and Development of Spiritual Consciousness,* in which she gives us some fairly extensive and detailed guidelines. Although her language was well-suited for her day and for those on a spectrum that ranges from those mildly interested in mysticism to college professors, it is often difficult to follow. Fortunately, there is a more recent perspective on the subjects of mysticism, mystic characteristics, and the mystic path, in Wayne Teasdall's, *The Mystic Heart* (1999).

Many people believe they have had at least one mystical experience in their lives. According to the nineteenth-century American psychologist and philosopher, William James, such singular experiences are identified by four general characteristics, namely,

1. They are more to do with feeling than intellect and cannot be conveyed using ordinary language

2. They have a noetic quality that manifests as a state of awareness beyond linear thinking.*

3. They transcend linear time, but rarely last more than a few moments.

4. They involve a state of passivity in the subject, as if the subject was 'swept up' and held safely by a supreme presence, not unlike an out-of–the-body experience.*

*As used in this context, the term 'noetic' refers to states of knowledge that are beyond the ordinary intellect.

However, there is a huge difference between the singular experience and identifying oneself *as being on the mystic path*. While the mystic path includes *some* of the general characteristics stated above which pertain to a single mystical experience, the reality is that it includes a great deal more. The mystic pilgrim is engaged in an ongoing process of travelling a very long and arduous path. Along this, there are certain markers or characteristics of identification. First, however, let us look at the larger view of the path.

According to both Underhill and Teasdall, the mystic pilgrim experiences distinctive states of consciousness and ways of being. Moreover, the path is one that is practical and active. The mystic participates in his–her process that is beneficial to the ongoing soul-growth. This aspect can feel familiar to us when we work with Bach's remedies, as the remedies themselves gently prompt us to engage in participation, reflection, awareness, and growth along our own soul-path. The mystical path is an experiential one. In other words, those on this path are in contact with what is ultimately real, according to Teasdall. A mystic *lives* his/her path,; he or she does not just *talk* about it. This is another way of reiterating Bodhidharma's 'all know the way, few walk it' (see Chapter Two). In addition, like the singular mystical experience, there are moments of awareness that lack sufficient descriptive language, but are implicit through a different way of knowing. Furthermore, the mystic experiences a knowing that is noetic, giving one 'direct knowledge of the ultimate reality or the Divine … a tasting knowledge of God'*

*Harper's Encyclopedia of Mystical and Paranormal Experience, p 384. *Teasdall, p. 23.

For the mystic, there is illumination of a universal connection between the temporal and cosmic world that does not require proof or explanation; it is integrative, absolute …. it simply is. Finally, Teasdall tells us that mystic spirituality is a practical, spiritual wisdom. In addition, within this wisdom there is particular knowledge of cosmic law and its process. The intuitive knowledge of this wisdom connects to the Divine at deep levels, and for some there is the added gift of sensing the emotions and motives of others when they are on their own journey.

The path which the mystic treads manifests in many forms, expressions and traditions. There are specific characteristics that identify the mystic and the mystical path. By referring to these characteristics as touchstones, we have the opportunity to weed out any charlatans lurking in our own particular bushes. At the same time, we can come to understand why Bach was a mystic.

Spiritual teachings, teachers, and scholars identify characteristics that are broadly-applied across many traditions and philosophies. However, because there are countless portrayals of mystics through the ages, we find that there is a collage that cuts across boundaries both sacred and secular alike. Mystical characteristics are to some extent subjective. Therefore not all 'mystics' will adhere to a precise list of identifiers, nor do all mystics exhibit mystical characteristics in the same fashion.

In her book, *Florence Nightingale, Mystic, Visionary, Healer,* Barbara Dossey notes that western mystics and saints did not live idyllic lives. The same, of course, is true for mystics of the East. According to Dossey, western mystics for the

most part lived a story that was complex and often full of
both external and internal chaos. This is because 'most of
these chosen and talented individuals took up the cause of
reform.'* When we look at profiles of other mystics, we see
that they lived lives characterized by selfless service, compassion, a form of spiritual practice, and far-reaching vision.
These mystical profiles from the past provide us with an interesting mixture of characteristics described by Underhill,
Teasdall and Dossey. The mix includes both balanced and
unbalanced aspects of their lives that brought them face to
face with difficult relationships. Many had a skewed sense
of self and doubted their abilities. While these struggles were
part of their fabric, mystics seem to have an overriding mo-
tivation that is or was a burning desire to achieve direct
knowledge of the Divine, both internally and externally. It
is the combination of such characteristics that ignited the
soul's fire in these individuals, propelling them onto the
mystic path.

Christian mystics such as Hildegard of Bingen (1098–
1179), St Teresa of Avila (1515–1582) and St John of the Cross
(1532–1591) exhibited a sense of compassion, unconditional
love and kindness for all living beings. These characteristics
often belong to mystics. However, within the framework of
their religious lifestyles, the manner in which they actively
manifested their visions differed as widely as their personal
stories.

Hildegard of Bingen, a feminist for her day, experienced
religious visions from early childhood in the way that many
of us commonly imagine make the mystic. With a confi-

*Dossey, p 425.

dence that can only come through a developed self-knowledge, she championed the place of women as being equal to that of men. Her writings and travels were prolific until her death in her early eighties in the twelfth century, and it is through writings that she criticized several of the major religions, including the doctrines of her own faith. With a vigorous interest in medicine, she 'integrated the four-element, four-humour natural healing system with spiritual wisdom'.* Is it such a coincidence that we see a similar philosophy in Edward Bach some seven hundred and fifty years later?

While St Teresa expressed her vision through numerous writings and the founding of seventeen strict convents, she seems to have been at odds with acceptance of self. As with many inhabitants of the ancient nunneries, St Teresa suffered from 'holy' anorexia, the practice of self-starvation, believing it to be a direct pathway to the Divine. Teresa 'regularly used an olive twig to induce vomiting so that she might receive the host without fear of rejecting it.'† In Teresa's case, as was the case for so many women coerced to a life within the cloister, there was a belief that the purer the body the more acceptable to the Divine. Sadly, this misguided belief masked the dynamics of shame-based guilt. This belief compounded the sense that they had virtually no control over their lives, and thus, they turned to their bodies, the only element these women could control in a male-driven culture.

A contemporary of and frequent correspondent with St Teresa, St John of the Cross expressed his mysticism through

*Harper's Encyclopedia of Mystical and Paranormal Experience, p 262. †Bell, p. 18.

prolific writings that focused on the 'soul's mystical journey toward God' through three stages of mystical union:
purgation, illuminations, and union. John's history tells us
that he firmly believed that suffering and detachment were
prerequisites for this union. Some say that he coined the
phrase, 'the dark night of the soul', which is presently used
to describe a state of intense personal struggle and, not so
coincidentally, describes the contracted emotional state of
Bach's remedy, Sweet Chestnut.

Just as the mystical path can manifest through various
behaviours, the initial mystical awakening can occur in a
variety of ways. Igniting the soul's fire can happen through
a singular event, or it may unfold through a process culmi-
nating in an eventual awareness of internal conflict with the
external environment. Taking a departure from these his-
torical Christian mystics, we can look to Florence Nightingale (1820–1879) and Swami Rama of the Himalayas
(1925–1997) as examples of contemporary mystics. Along
with tribal Shamans, Yogis, Buddhists, Cabbalists, Sufis and
countless others who make up the mystic consortium from
diverse traditions, these two individuals hold fast their own
places on the mystic register. While both came from wealth,
their agendas of selfless service to humanity were as diverse
as their cultural backgrounds.

Florence Nightingale's initial experience occurred
through a singular event. Like Hildegard of Bingen and
France's fifteenth-century Joan of Arc, Florence Nightingale
'received a Call from God to be of service' when she was
only sixteen, on February 7, 1837. From then on, Nightingale, in spite of chronic and severe physical maladies

throughout her lifetime, struggled to pursue a vision and mission dedicated to medical and social reform. Despite her comfortable upbringing, she did not live a life of simplicity or one of privacy.

Driven by her passion and fire to achieve Divine Union with the Absolute, Florence Nightingale was clearly an agent of change. She devoted her life to revolutionizing the sanitation methods used in British hospitals; she pushed for reform of the British Military's healthcare system and the elevation of the nursing profession. All of this activity required her to be very much in the world. She clearly had macrocosmic vision, and it was through these outward and very worldly manifestations of her desire that she evidently attained a level of union with the Divine in the last years of her life: 'the longings of my heart accomplished—and now drawn to Thee by difficulties and disappointments. Homeward bound, I have entered in.'* According to Underhill, the two women who left the deepest mark on military history in England and France, Nightingale and Joan d' Arc, were women driven by mystical compulsion.

Although born to a learned Brahmin family in the eastern Indian province of Uttar Pradesh, Swami Rama spent his youth living in the foothills of the Himalayas, where a yogi and saint of Bengal raised him. His early education took place in the monasteries of the Himalayas, where he learned the disciplines of yoga, science and philosophy. Here he studied with other spiritual adepts, including Mahatma Gandhi, Sri Aurobindo, and Rabindranath Tagore. In the early 1950s, he spent eleven months sealed in a six-by-four cave with

*Dossey, p. 425.

only a single pinpoint of light. There he engaged in an intense state of meditation and the yoga practice of Pranayama, or control of the breath. At the end of the eleven months, he emerged with a life-vision for himself, which was one of serving humanity.

In this service, his goal was to teach others how to access the 'teacher within'; and his life from then on focused on bringing the sacred teachings of the Himalaya to the West. Furthermore, these teachings had their foundation in his vast knowledge of medicine, psychology, parapsychology and philosophy. In 1971, he founded the Himalayan International Institute of Yoga Science and Philosophy in the United States saying, 'We must build a centre of life which will be an important bridge between East and West.'* As a result, his vision continues to thrive globally through various channels promoted by his followers and devotees.

While at first glance Edward Bach may not appear to be a mystic, Teasdall states that 'each of us is called to be a mystic'.† This is most definitely a surprise. It a surprise in that each of us has such potential. It affords us, as well, the opportunity to perceive Bach in an entirely different light. In this, we have yet another surprise. This new perspective becomes important to our ability to embrace the core messages the flower remedies hold for our souls and the roles they play in igniting our soul's fire and purpose. As seekers, we are in a process of initiation that requires we travel down into the inner self. This is not an exercise of the head and mind that gravitates toward rationalization.

For this reason, the journey is not an easy one. Being

**http://www.himalayaninstitute.org/swamirama. †Teasdall, p. 119.

called to the mystic path, our soul-path becomes one of a
series of initiations. Initiations are

> *an expansion of consciousness to a realization of the all-ness and completeness
> and universality of God's love. That expansion of consciousness or initiation comes
> when you can . . . hold fast to faith—even if it seems that all you have worked
> and stood for, all you believe in and hope for, crashes and crumbles about you.
> Now is the very limit of your test, and your initiation is at hand. . . . When you
> are pushed to the very last degree of endurance, the light breaks for you and
> you know that all you have stood for and held to is eternal truth.* **

In other words, initiations are not meant to be easy.

In exploring Bach from this perspective, we can discover
the essence of this man beyond his gifts as a brilliant physician. Leaping into the new territory, we have the opportunity to witness an expression of absolute and contemporary
mysticism and in the process perhaps discover mystical characteristics within ourselves.

A pattern that seems to appear with most mystics is that
they disconnect, in a sense, from a life that has been familiar. How and when this disconnection takes place varies in-
dividually. For many the driving force is an inner struggle
between the incessant chatter of the rational mind and listening to the voice of the soul. As Bach began his work with
the remedies, he identified this conflict as the cause of illness and disease.

Not unlike the behavioural patterns of other mystics,
Bach's obsession with work clearly intensified the chronic
fragility of his health. He added further demands upon himself when he chose to live a simple life after he left London.
At first glance, the decision would seem to have been a sup-

---

*White Eagle, in *Stella Polaris*, 1952–3, p. 184.

portive one in view of his other behaviours. However, this was not the case. This choice led to very difficult circumstances far different from the financial freedom he had enjoyed throughout his consulting practice in London. When he and Nora Weeks left London to continue and expand the work with the remedies, Bach refused to charge patients for his services. As a result, his resources were chronically scarce: so much so that when they settled at Mt Vernon (the Bach Centre today), Bach had to make most of the furniture for his consulting rooms himself.*

Solitude is an environment that most mystics crave. Bach was no exception, in that his relationships (both personal and professional) seemed to fluctuate. While Nora Weeks reports that he liked to go to the pub for a singsong and a few pints with the lads, information regarding close friends away from his work is not available from her. During his marriage to his first wife, Bach fathered a child by another woman, whom he later married after his first wife died of diphtheria. He later separated from his second wife, in 1922.†

Clearly, Bach was an enigma. On the one hand, both Weeks and Barnard describe him as a man who could be blunt, impatient, and yet unendingly compassionate. Weeks comments that while he had a keen interest in village affairs he needed unending time to be alone and to walk the countryside. Progressively abandoned by the profession that had just a few years previously held him in the highest esteem, it seems that the company he most preferred was that of his Masonic brothers and his few companions who were working with him in the remedy research.

*Weeks, *Discoveries, p.* 111. †Barnard, p.305.

The need for solitude among those on the mystic path, such as Bach, carries a double-edged sword. Solitude can evolve into intense loneliness and crisis of spirit as the individual becomes faced with his or her own dragons and the abyss. Dossey reports that Nightingale entered into her 'dark night of the soul' (one of the phases of spiritual development), following her 'intense work on Harley Street, in the Crimean War, and on (her work for) army medical reform. Her chronic ill health combined with stress, overexertion, and the deaths of her soul-mates ... brought her to a low point until she realized that God was taking all human help away from her 'in order to compel me to lean on Him alone.'*

Aside from grappling with the mystic's emblematic characteristics of chronic health problems, difficult relationships, the desire for simplicity of life, and the experience of intense loneliness, it is Bach's unique rapport with nature that underscores the fact of his walking the path of a natural or nature mystic. The Divine has produced many natural or 'nature mystics' according to Teasdall, who has quite a lot to say about their characteristics. As a group, nature mystics have an intrinsic connection to all of life through the natural world. For them there is an innate understanding of the symbology and messages nature freely offers to humankind. For the nature mystic this connection to the natural world is a 'reality [that] is revelational ... that trigger[s] higher states of awareness.'†

In other words, there is an intimate relationship and, most importantly, a level of consciousness with the Divine

*Dossey, p. 425. †Teasdall. p. 192.

through the natural world that simply does not resonate to such depths with others. Nature mystics express these dynamics through mediums such as the arts, ritual, writing, and the arts of medicine and healing. Edward Bach expressed his symbiotic relationship with nature and his service to humanity through the discovery of the remedies and his passionate desire that others freely learn how to use them for their wellbeing and discovery of soul-purpose.

On the mystic path, there is no room for greed, arrogance, or over-concern with accruing substantial possessions as a means of identity or power. If these emotions become driving forces, the conscious awareness of and the connection to all life, along with the ability to feel the struggle and pain of others, is unattainable. Some pilgrims on the mystic path also possess the extraordinary gift of high sensitivity to the motives and emotional depths of others. Edward Bach is included in this group. As Bach's intuitive abilities became increasingly stronger, he had the ability to heal by touch and, on occasion, had the ability to foretell events. Weeks notes:

Through his finely developed sense of touch he was able to feel the vibrations and power emitted by any plant he wished to test; and so greatly was his body receptive to these vibrations that it reacted instantaneously. If he held the petal or bloom of some plant in the palm of his hand or placed it on his tongue, he would feel in his body the effects of the properties within that flower. *

Bach's great compassion and links with all things and people formed a link between them and him, and by reason of this sympathy, he would hear the call for help from any in distress. †

This awareness is essential for one on the mystic path and

*Weeks, Discoveries, p. 50.   †Weeks, *Discoveries*, pp. 106–7.

for those of us attempting to discover our soul-purpose. However, this does not mean that there are not struggles, obstacles, and disillusionment along the way. According to Bach's friend and colleague, Dr. F. J. Wheeler, 'the last seven years of his [Bach's] life were lonely ones for him; his work, during that period was based entirely on the knowledge that he gained intuitively and for such, the world has little understanding or encouragement, needing causes, scientific provings, before it is ready to believe.'* From statements made in one of his last public appearances before his death, it is evident that Bach had found solace in and connection to the Divine through his work with the remedies. He said:

> We carry a Spark of the Divine, that within us resides a Vital and Immortal Principle. And the more that Spark of Divinity shines within us, the more our lives radiate Its sympathy, Its compassion and Its love, the more we are beloved by our fellow-men.... From time immemorial, man has looked at two great sources for Healing. To his Maker, and to the Herbs of the field, which his Maker has placed for the relief of those who suffer. Yet one Truth has mostly been forgotten. That those Herbs of the field placed for Healing, by comforting, by soothing, by relieving our cares, our anxieties, bring us nearer to the Divinity within. And it is that increase of the Divinity within which heals us.†

Furthermore, spiritual teachings stress, 'Humanity is one vast brotherhood of life; that all nature is part of you—you are part of nature'.§ The portrait of Edward Bach as a mystic is one that brings into focus some compelling realities about the man. In our contemplation, we come to realize that were he alive today, his compassion would undeniably reach out

---

*Weeks, *Discoveries*, p. 139. †Masonic Lecture, 1936, in Barnard, *Collected Writings*. §White Eagle, *White Eagle on the Great Spirit*, p. 75.

to us. Whether physician or friend, acquaintance or not, he would sit beside us, hold our hand and encourage us through our distress. He would stand at our back as we face difficult challenges and he would be healing us with his insights, energy, and his remedies.

While Dr Bach is no longer with us, his messages are. Exploration of our emotions is a necessity for discovery of our soul's fire if we are serious about travelling our mystical path. As we acknowledged back in Chapter One, this exploration is a formidable challenge. Most of us will attempt to negotiate our way around what is actually a prerequisite for our work, convincing ourselves that confronting the dragons of our emotions is not only unnecessary, it promises very unpleasant experiences.

Nevertheless, this confrontation is essential. In the chapters that follow, we shall be taking a closer look at the ways in which our personal dragons manifest and how we can transform them from adversaries into elements of empowerment.

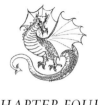

CHAPTER FOUR

HERE BE DRAGONS

MEDIEVAL cartographers had a common practice of mapping the world as they knew it. When the mapmaker had ascertained all he could from his storehouse of knowledge on geography, he would letter the phrase, *'Here be Dragons'*, across the void thus creating a boundary between the safety of territory that was known, and the ominous abyss of the unknown beyond. Throughout our lifetime, the Divine pushes us through dark tunnels and just when we think we may be seeing the light at the end, we emerge, only to find that we are looking into the abyss … where the dragons lurk. And yet, it is this confrontation of sorts that signals our initiation onto the mystic path in our quest to discover our soul-purpose.

The image of the dragon was a familiar one to the ancients and in the present, it still is. The national symbol of Wales is the icon of a Red Dragon, while a moment's thought of the dragon also conjures up Scotland's eternally-famous water dragon, 'Nessie'. Some sources of Welsh mythology connect dragons to the four elements of fire, air, water and earth and for us as we travel on our journey, it is these elemental dragons of emotion that hold keys to our own unexplored territory. It is this very territory we need to ex-

plore because that which ignites our soul's fire also lights
the way upon our soul or mystic path that is waiting for us
in the emotional territory of our primeval great deep. It is
this excavation that will assist us in moving through the
baptism of fire, air, water, earth, and which will move us
forward upon our path.

Draig-Teine*
I Am on Fire with Passion, Obsession and Pain

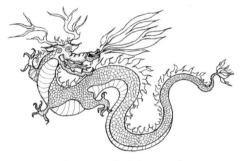

In astrology, mythology, and alchemy fire is synonymous
with energy, mastery and, most importantly, transmutation.
The emotions of passion, obsession and pain in one way or
another are emotions that herald our initiation through the
element of fire. The Universe and everything within it works
within a framework of polarities, including the realms of
science and spirit. As both scientist and mystic, Edward Bach
recognized the polarities of emotions in his patients and particularly within himself. The foundation of his work with
the Remedies is built upon the realization that the negative
or contracted state of emotions fuel illness and disease and
that trading contraction for expansion is the only way to

*Draig-Teine, Draig-Uisge, Draig-Talamh and Draig-Athar, are sometimes
represented as the dragons of fire, water, earth and air in Welsh lore.

wholeness and growth. But, in order to shift our relationships with toxic emotions, which he *knew* only too well from
his own life, we must be willing and have the courage to
confront our emotional dragons head-on.

For most of us, the emotion of passion conjures up positive images such as the pleasant feelings that one experiences
in the ardour of love or in the enthusiasm for art or music.
Years ago, when I was an undergraduate, a professor of mine
in comparative religions made the statement, 'whatever
your passion is, that which means the most to you, this is
your religion'. For some time I never could understand his
thought-process fully, until I realized that he was talking
about emotion.

The emotion of passion in the positive sense is exciting,
stimulating, and can take your breath away. The work toward a universal ideal often gives birth to passion because of
the felt passion for the cause which, when balanced, creates
leaders and teachers for the good of humanity. However,
when the fire of such passion converts into the contracted
negative state, it becomes so intense that the qualities of lead-
ership and wisdom become zealous, wilful, and inflexible,
burning out the individual and burning those around them.
Sadly, we see such contracted passion all too vividly in the
world today in which the original spirit has become intan-
gible and lost.

In our passion, anxiety appears. It can ratchet up to a state
of obsession—which can make us believe that we will never
have enough, do enough, or be enough. In our perception
that there will never be enough, we begin to want and grasp
for more. This grasping, Buddhist psychologist Jack Korn-

field comments, is driven by the need to feed the chronic wanting within us, which he identifies as our 'hungry ghost'.* If only we had more, could do more, we would *be more*. It is ironic that in our frenzied obsession to feed our ghost, we come to believe that the fire of our intensity will correspond to progress on our soul-path. What we do not comprehend is that the fire of the contracted emotional obsession burns so hot that it forestalls any movement forward on our path. This is not the fire of positive emotions that ignites our soul-purpose. Instead, the smoke from our obsessive fire dragon billows around us and we are unable to see our intended path. While we are unable to see or recognize that we shall never be able to fill our 'hungry ghost', our wanting continues out of control, whispering to us that there will never be enough. And, we never will have enough … unless we can shift our perspective.

When we put our hands too close to the fire we feel pain. A woman in labour, about to give birth, feels pain with the growing intensity of each contraction. Contraction brings pain whether it is physical or emotional. From an emotional perspective, it can be some time before we experience the painful outcome of this fire; but when we do, it always comes with the strings of karmic law and the law of correspondence attached. The good news is that in the excavation of our emotional 'dig' we have the opportunity to engage the positive nature of the fire dragon, which can manifest as constructive energy and mastery. Above all, fire transmutes, purifies, and transforms … and in spiritual law, *Love* is the elemental lesson of *Fire.*†

*Kornfield, *A Path with Heart*, 1993. †White Eagle, *The Path of the Soul*, pp. 73-4.

Draig-Athar
I am suspended in air from restlessness,
confusion and with detachment

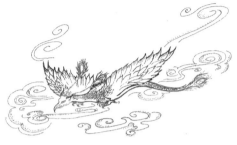

The element air is a metaphysical symbol for inspiration, insight and, in its highest expression, illumination. These are all characteristics of the mystic path; but for some, the fullest and most balanced expression of these markers is out of reach when we become mired in detachment, confusion and restlessness. It is in these states of *non-awareness* that we circumvent our soul's agenda for our journey.

Recalling that the initiations we experience on our soul-path are not meant to be easy, cosmic law challenges us by propelling us out of our comfort zones. These 'opportunities' show up not once, but on numerous occasions, pushing us into uncharted space that shows up through a variety of manifestations. In these moments, when anxiety sets in and we lose our footing, the dragon of air takes up residence in the seat of our emotional self and life can become scary. The experience makes us feel as if we are flying at high altitudes, deprived of the necessary oxygen to maintain our focus. In this space we panic, certain that we are losing our way on the journey. Reactively, we grasp for safety in the mind and in our anxiety and restlessness, we count on the rational brain taking over and getting things under control. This is illusion.

The reality is that if we were able to acknowledge our denial concerning the true state of our emotions, we would be able to admit that in fact we don't know who we are or where we really are going. However, since we cannot do this when we are in the clutches of the Air Dragon, we mask our disorientation by appearing indifferent and detached to the rest of the world. The difficulty is that we are not able to hold this space indefinitely because eventually our soul will shatter this illusion through chaos in one form or another.

Emotional betrayals that lead to loss of faith within our self and with others are often the driving force behind personal chaos. The irony is that from the spiritual level, those who feel they have been betrayed, and then lose faith in self and those around them, are often the people who possess deep wisdom garnered from many lifetimes of experience and learning. And while they may sense something urging them to speak from deep within, there may be a vague sense of some unidentified trauma that keeps them from pursuing, much less expressing, this intuitive sense or *soul-voice.* Since they cannot specifically identify this vague sensation, they dismiss it and the struggle continues. The rational mind becomes insistent that these individuals 'keep a lid on it', deferring any notions of intuition for the mind to sort out. For those who are caught in this impasse on the mystic path and unable to trust, much less speak, their intuitive voice with confidence, the internal struggle intensifies and the wisdom that is held within the soul remains obscured. On the brink of internal chaos, they seek refuge by detaching from the external environment and thus escaping upwards into the ethers of the mind. From this space, there are essentially two ways of being. If the individual goes one way, he or she rationalizes everything, including his or her emotions, speaking of them as if they were something viewed under a microscope at arms' length. If the individual goes the other, he or she takes on the 'air' of being 'in the world, but not of it'.

From an energetic perspective, the inherent danger is that in either scenario, these individuals have become ungrounded. In this state, a door opens which invites an entirely new way of being in the world that is not on the soul's agenda. Either these individuals completely retreat into the perceived safety of introversion, or they develop a skewed sense of self-important grandiosity.

For those with illusions of grandeur, fantasies of extraordinary 'spiritual gifts' place them in an imagined position of power over 'less-evolved' individuals. The journey of the path, as the Buddhists say, is simple; 'chop wood, carry water'. But for those who live in the realm of fantasy about themselves and their 'gifts', they simply do not plug into the reality of the journey. Conversely, for those truly on the mystic path, like Edward Bach, the spiritual agenda really is to 'chop wood, carry water.' Sadly, in the approaching Aquarian Age, we are so inundated with self-professed gurus, psychics, clairvoyants, shamans and mystics, that it is difficult to discern the wheat from the chaff. However, spiritual teachings tell us 'most major work is done quietly'. Bach knew this as well. He pursued his work with the rem-

*Original Writings, p. 176.

edies without pretence and in a steadfast manner that did not engage fanfare and notoriety. His was a system of healing that he identified as 'simple and pure'.* So in our effort to discover what ignites our soul's fire, progress on our path becomes measured by our level of self-awareness and the ability to tap into and trust the innate wisdom of our soul-voice. When this happens, it brings with it moments of grounded insight, inspiration, and ultimately, wise illumination that we are meant to share selflessly with others along the way. This is the soul's intent for each of us, for the lesson of the element *Air* is *Brotherhood*.

Draig-Uisge
I am drowning in the waters of fear, anger and grief

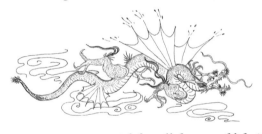

The element water, essential for all forms of life 'Creates, nourishes and destroys physical form .... [it] is concerned with the soul of things—with the psychic aspect of our being, that part of us which senses, reflects, and absorbs the impressions of the world around us'.*

Classically, the element of water symbolizes emotions dwelling in the very root of our being. And, like a body of water, these emotions can be calm. Conversely, the water dragon of our emotions can suddenly rise up from the

*Joan Hodgson, *Astrology the Sacred Science*, p. 62.

depths of our being manifesting in emotions that churn, sending us out of control.

As a mystic who possessed the gift of being able to intuit unspoken emotional states of others, Edward Bach felt the emotional dragons of fear, anger, and grief from those around him. In view of this, it is no coincidence that his earliest flower remedies were ones that address these particular contracted emotional states.

When we experience fear in its positive manifestation, it functions as a necessary safety-net warning us of danger, cautioning us to stop so that we may reassess our situation, behaviour, or plan of action. However, irrational and unrestrained fear catapults us out of emotional balance, driving us into watery depths that results in destructive behaviour and unwise choices. Fear of loss, the emotion that is one of our most intrinsic, can drive us into depression, non-action and disempowerment.

There is no authentic spiritual philosophy that promises the mystic path to our soul's purpose will be easy. In fact, quite the opposite is true; and facing our fears can be guaranteed to be a prerequisite for forward progress. Quite simply, there is no way around this one; either you face your fear or you don't. Spiritual teachings also tell us that if we dwell on those things we are most afraid of, we will draw them to ourselves in one form or another just so that we will have the opportunity to transcend and transmute those fears. In other words, the only way to get to the other side of fear is to go through it. If we find that we simply are unable to master such opportunities this lifetime, not to worry; the Universe has the ability to supply endless opportunities for lifetimes to come. Such is the way of the *laws of karma and rebirth.*

Difficult as it is, the emotion that holds the greatest power over us is psychological fear. The path of the mystic includes service; it is this path that is taking us into the Aquarian age of universal unity. Each of us possesses the potential to be a mystic. Fear, within a heartbeat, is *the* one contracted emotion that can abort our dreams for fulfilling such a destiny. A familiar bedfellow of fear is the dragon of anger, for usually it is fear that fuels the anger. Anger can bear many facets, including rage. While the experience of fear can have a beneficial effect, as in warning us of danger, there is no benefit to rageful or revengeful anger or the behaviour that it drives. 'In-your-face rage' is an all-too-common way of being these days and is one that has gone from a microcosmic framework into a macrocosmic explosion with terrifying global repercussions.

But anger is not always 'in-your-face rage'. The smouldering emotion of repressed anger is just as destructive. This emotional state can remain banked like coals of a fire for years, ready to reignite at any given moment. Bach identified this type of anger as one that leads to resentment, self-pity and bitterness. As secondary emotions, they set the stage for the eternal victim, who in his–her unrealized state of entitlement is merely another aborted mystic.

The emotional dragon of anger, whether it is rageful or repressed, harms others physically and psychologically. In addition, it eventually turns in on the self, destroying the cellular structure. The body cannot tolerate this kind of pressure indefinitely and if these dragons are not quelled through resolution and balance, the body will break down. We can, in what seems to be a heartbeat, be brought to our knees through illness or through acute mental stress or distress. This is the point at which we shall either have the opportunity to find resolution and rebuild our health, or we shall not. If not, resuming my earlier metaphor, there will always be the next train, leaving the station in the next incarnation.

There is yet another water dragon that can drown us, and it is the dragon of grief. Grief involves loss of anything that is dear to us, has provided safety to us, or has been a part of us. While it is a natural part of life, it is not an emotion that our soul means for us to experience perpetually on our path. The experience of grief is to teach us the process of honouring and then letting go. It is part of the constant expansion process. As we honour the process and move through it, we create space for the energy of new experiences and opportunities to present themselves. And it is in this constant movement that we experience growth; exactly what our soul intends for us.

In her many writings and workshops, Caroline Myss often refers to those who become married to their grief as 'staying in their woundology'. I have also heard her comment, when referring to former clients of hers that they could stay in their woundology as long as they wished; she simply was not staying there with them. Myss' point here is that staying stuck in our grief is a guaranteed way to stay stuck in life and, therefore, stuck on our mystic path. This does not mean that we should not honour our grief as a necessary process of the human experience, but in order to make progress in discovering our soul-purpose, we have to be willing to let go of the grief and move on. Nothing is indefinite in the human experience and grief shouldn't be either. Grief is the messenger of change and with change, there is opportunity. The issue is, how will we respond to our opportunities?

If we stay stuck in our fear, our anger, our rage or our grief we will not learn the elemental lesson of *Water*, which is *Peace*.

Draig-Talamh
I am bound to the earth by resistance,
indecision and worldly fears

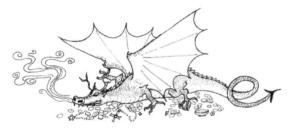

In spiritual teachings, esoteric writings and psychology, reference to 'being grounded' (or ungrounded, as the case may be) often appears. In these contexts, the concept of 'being grounded or ungrounded' is a description of the energetic or emotional state of an individual. Often it refers to both simultaneously. The inference in these descriptions is that the individual is well-balanced emotionally and energetically, able to perceive his or her surrounding environment with clear perception. But as with all things, there can be too much of a good thing and the element earth is no exception; we can be far too entrenched in the ground. The expression, 'earthbound' is not one that refers to a positive state of affairs. When seen in older writings, it refers to the soul or spirit of a dear, but expired, Aunt Petunia or Uncle Herald who is not able to ascend into the glory of the ethers.

As we proceed along our mystic path, our environment constantly changes, and there are times when we become excessively grounded in the element earth. Whether we are aware of it or not (and often we are just simply oblivious), we find ourselves at an impasse. Here the dragon of earth has captured us, manifesting as excessive resistance, indecision and/or our old nemesis—fear.

If we reflect thoughtfully on the emotion of fear, it is not difficult to see that as a basic emotion it pushes the 'buttons' that ignite many secondary, contracted emotions that are part of the human condition. If we recall the contracted emotional states of the fire, air and water dragons, we can easily see that fear is a primary emotion. The contracted experience of the element earth is no exception, although it appears through different expressions.

Emotional resistance is very powerful and refers to a state of emotional contraction that prevents us from 'hearing' valuable advice and urgings from those around us. But, far more important to our spiritual journey, resistance prevents us from hearing critical *messages from our soul.* An axiom of spiritual law dictates that the more we resist, the harder the lesson. Furthermore, that which we resist the most is actually the thing we need to embrace. But, do we listen? *Of course not.*

Esoteric astrologers often look at the influence and aspects of the planet Pluto in a chart in order to determine those areas of an individual's life or behaviour that might prove disruptive to their soul-growth. Astrologically referred to as 'the destroyer', Pluto is often referred to as the 'cosmic two-by-four', in the sense of a heavy wooden joist. Prior to what astrologers call a 'Pluto transit', we typically are given many clues and opportunities by the Universe to make changes in our lives that are necessary if we are to proceed on our path. Unfortunately for us, we continue on, believing we know better than anyone or anything how we should do this journey of ours. When we ignore such opportunities, the result is a 'Pluto transit' that takes no prisoners, and we are forced to make changes. Furthermore, strange as it may seem, there appears to be a direct correlation between the extent of our resistance to change and the intensity of our particular experience. Sometimes we just do not get it until we are hit over the head.

Indecision is a bedfellow of resistance. In our resistance, life does not fall into place as we think it should (because, remember, we aren't listening or paying attention), so we become full of self-doubt and eventually move into a chronic state of indecisiveness. There is not one decision that we can make with a steadfast mind and, as a result, we forever question ourselves, coming to a point wherein no decision is *the* decision.

Unlike some of our other emotions that possess positive attributes which balance their contracted states, neither resistance or indecisiveness have any positive value. Stuck in a place that has us trapped by these two emotional contractors, there is no way we can possibly move forward on our mystic path, much less discover what will ignite our soul's fire.

As if resistance and indecision were not enough, the culprit often lurking behind these two states of being is fear of worldly things. These are the things Edward Bach described as the fears of every day life* If we are afraid of the dark, of illness, pain, being with others ... the world in general, is it any wonder that trapped in the clutches of the earth dragon of our worldly fears we become resistant and indecisive? Sadly, being irrationally afraid of the environment around us, and being resistant and indecisive, prevents us from being in the world. In this state we are unable to reach out, to engage with others, to connect with our soul-purpose. In a phrase, we are unable to be of service, and the paradox in this is that the elemental lesson of *Earth* is *Service*.

As we journey along our mystical path in search of whatever ignites our soul fire and purpose, it is a given that we will encounter the emotional dragons of fire, air, water and earth. But what we need to remember is that along the way our soul is whispering to us, cautioning us to pay attention, to be aware, to reflect and to participate in slaying them.

*Barnard, *Collected Writings,* p. 37.

CHAPTER FIVE

IN THE NAME OF SERVICE
AND BROTHERHOOD:
THE TWELVE GREAT REMEDIES

As a mystic and student of the esoteric, Bach strongly believed that every one of us is Divine. And in our Divinity, each of us has a job to do in this lifetime in the name of service and brotherhood. This is our soul-path, our mystical path. Whether or not we achieve our goal in this lifetime is uncertain. What is certain is that according to cosmic law we are given plenty of opportunity for discovering what ignites our soul's fire, either in this incarnation, or in future ones.

In earlier chapters, there was discussion regarding the missteps some people tend to make in their desire to be spiritual. Ignoring the emotional excavations that must be a part of walking the mystical or soul-path, some of us choose to focus upon our sacred shopping, anxiously obsessed that we will miss the spiritual train. In making misguided choices through our obsessions and anxieties, we tend to become intransigent and dogmatic in our chosen beliefs and rituals in the name of spirituality. Unfortunately, in this mindset we can take on the undesirable mantle of pious self-righteousness. The danger here is that this attitude can lead to unwarranted cruelty, judgment, or anger towards others who are far from deserving of the repercussions of such misguided emotions.

The reality is that spirituality is not about piety or self-righteousness; it is about *service and brotherhood.* By working the patterns of our own feelings and shifting those that are contracted into an expansive state, we can make the discovery within ourselves of our own soul's fire. This divinity manifests in the simplicity of desire to serve without expectation. Divinity lies in the understanding of what 'brotherhood' truly means. In this understanding, Edward Bach was crystal-clear in his writings:

> *Impersonal service done, not even for spiritual promotion, but just for the desire to serve. This is the keynote of the hindrances you are now to investigate.**

Bach was intrigued with the patterns of numbers, which is not surprising as Freemasonry has its roots in mathematics. He maintained that the keys to transforming our 'emotional hindrances', so that we may access our spiritual self, rests in the spiritual heart of twelve distinct soul-types or soul-personalities. Alongside these soul-types, he placed the first twelve of his remedies, those he identified as the Twelve Great Remedies', later calling them 'the Twelve Healers'.†

Clearly, while the universe may hold an infinite number of soul-types, Bach chose not to tackle the prospect of such a massive field and instead opted to keep his work simple within the twelve. He also maintained that these twelve soul-types comprised individual collectives, or groups, and that each of us belong to one of these 'soul-groups'. His message in all of this was

---

*Barnard, *Collected Writings*, pp. 15–16. †Barnard, 2002, pp. 140–41. From this point in the book, the Twelve Great Remedies will be referred to as the Twelve Healers.

that our own spiritual responsibility, along with that of our companions in the group, is about transformation.

By working through the hindrance or soul-lesson of our particular soul-collective we have the opportunity to realize its 'virtue'. Thus, by engaging in the process of our soul's lesson, we each carry out our responsibility of imparting its particular virtue to the rest of humanity.* For each of us, this is *our service for all humankind, which is brotherhood in the widest sense.* In our soul-work, the Twelve Healers themselves are agents of connection and change, for they shift the place of our consciousness from selfishness to selflessness. Further, in our 'work', we can think of the soul-hindrances identified by Bach as contracted (negative) soul-states and conversely the virtues as expanded (positive) soul-states. This exemplar is in perfect harmony with the universe from the perspective of both science and spirit. In all of nature, science works in polarities and in parallels and so does the spiritual plane:

> *We would draw your attention to the importance of balance. These two aspects, light and dark, positive and negative, are working together to bring about balance and equilibrium, which is one of the fundamental laws of life. The ultimate is absolute balance within the microcosm, and within the macrocosm.†*

In the process of walking our mystical path, awareness brings us to discover that contracted emotions can lead us into a place of self-absorption and illusion. The reality is that in this space it is impossible for us to offer service, much less take on this responsibility in the spirit of global brotherhood. It is from this perspective that Bach believed that if we can

*Barnard, 2002, p. 139. †White Eagle, *White Eagle on the Great Spirit,* p. 46.

identify our soul-lesson (by way of the soul-profiles of his Twelve Healers) we have the opportunity for transformation. It is through this transformation that we discover what ignites our soul's fire. Once we make this discovery, we are better able to move forward on our mystical path of service and brotherhood.

While Bach has a great deal to say on this subject, it is important for us to keep in mind, and have appreciation for, the fact that he himself was on a path of continual soul-growth and awareness. As a true mystic and healer, Edward Bach had the ability to facilitate the connection between his mind and intuitive heart, but this does not mean that his path was clear or easy. As his understanding and intuitive abilities deepened, he made modifications in some details and impressions concerning the remedies as a system of healing.

While there are slight variances in his philosophical language depending on the audience he was addressing and his own level of awareness, the essential spirit of his message remains constant. That message is that, at their foundation, the Twelve Healers are soul-medicine, capable of providing light into the hidden corners of a person's soul. They provide a bridge of light between the soul and our conscious awareness, bringing the wisdom held safely within the intuitive heart upwards into our reality. In *Some Fundamental Considerations of Disease and Cure,* Bach writes, referring to the highest class of plants and their healing qualities as having 'the power to elevate our vibrations, and thus draw down spiritual power, which cleanses mind and body, and heals.'* However, Bach also recognized that there was more involved in the issue of illness and disease than an individual being

able to identify their soul-lesson. He concluded that we exhibit 'mood states' and chronic personality characteristics
on the mundane level as well. In this awareness, he recognized that mood states and personality characteristics could
preclude the discovery of our soul-type. In addition, they
directly affect our state of health. Thus, the successful treatment of illness depends upon identifying the mood states
and/or personality characteristics. He believed that contracted moods and personality characteristics could be so
entrenched within us that until these are addressed and
brought into a state of balance, one cannot possibly identify
the soul-type and its lesson with any accuracy.†

Bach first wrote of this realization in *The Twelve Healers and
Four Helpers.* In this book he further describes the four additional remedies that he thought of as adjuncts or helpers.
This group later evolved into a total of seven to complete
the first nineteen of the thirty-eight Bach remedies. However, throughout his work, Bach maintained that our foundation is anchored in our soul-type and the lesson that it is
meant to learn and teach.

To Bach's way of thinking, there was always something
new to learn, or something upon which to expand. As an
example, there is a variance in the language he used in *Free
Thyself.* In it Bach maintains '*there is no failure when you are doing
your utmost, whatever the apparent result*'.* Conversely, he uses the
term 'failing' and 'spiritual failings' in both his early descriptions of the first twelve remedies and in his later writings. In
addition to these descriptions, he seems to have also used the

---

*Barnard, *Collected Writings,* p. 161. †The issues of mood states and personality
types will be addressed in succeeding chapters. §Barnard, *Collected Writings,* p. 70.

words, 'qualities to develop' 'weakness' and 'soul-lessons' inter-
changeably in his writings. In any case, through what Barnard
identifies as 'the architecture of the twelve healers',† Bach laid
out the pattern of both the spiritual failings (hindrances,
weakness) and corresponding virtues (soul-lessons, qualities to develop) as they correspond to the remedies known
as the Twelve Healers in the context of soul-types:

Failing	Herb	Virtue
Fear	Mimulus	Sympathy
Weakness	Centaury	Strength
Doubt	Gentian	Understanding
Indecision	Scleranthus	Steadfastness
Ignorance	Cerato	Wisdom
Grief	Water Violet	Joy
Restraint	Chicory	Love
Indifference	Clematis	Gentleness
Terror	Rock Rose	Courage
Restlessness	Agrimony	Peace
Over-enthusiasm	Vervain	Tolerance
Impatience	Impatiens	Forgiveness

Clearly, each of Bach's soul-types also can reflect temporary emotional states or characteristics of an individual's personality. Leaving this acknowledgment aside, Bach's concept
of soul-types implies that a karmic soul-lesson is involved
for each type, and that in these lessons, there is an emphasis
on the need for a transformation. Furthermore, such transformations involve the complexities of expansion in their
height and depth of understanding.

*Barnard, *Collected Writings*, p. 107. †Barnard 2002, p. 137.

For those who have an interest in astrology, there is another facet to these early writings. As I stated earlier, Bach had more than a passing interest in a variety of esoteric subjects. It appears that one area of interest to him was that of astrology, thus accounting for his initially linking the Twelve Healers to the astrological position of the moon within the twelve signs of the zodiac:

> These types of personality are indicated to us by the moon according to which sign of the Zodiac she is in at birth, and a study of this will give us the following points: 1. The type of personality, 2. His [her] object and his [her] work in life, [and] 3. The remedy which will assist him [her] in that work. . . .
>
> Our personality we learn from the position of the moon at birth; our dangers of interference from the planets. . . . If we can hold our personality, be true unto ourselves we need fear no planetary or outside influence. The remedies assist us to maintain our personality. *

While it would make a fascinating study to follow Bach's life and soul-path through the science of astrology, that is not the focus intended here. I wish simply to point out Bach's initial intent in tying the twelve remedies to the zodiac. At the time, he believed that astrology provided a channel for discovering the soul's personality and its intended lessons through the place in the zodiac of the natal moon.

In Bach's own natal , or birth chart, the moment of his birth (September 25, 1886, 00:00:19 GMT), places a strong link between his natal Neptune (27° 40´ Taurus, in the Eleventh House) and his natal Sun (1°50´ Libra, very close to the Fourth House cusp). This particular link is one that astrologers often find in the charts of mystics. However, it is the zodiacal placing of his natal moon in this lifetime that gives

*Barnard, *Collected Writings*, pp. 77–8.

us clues to his soul-lesson and the path he was meant to travel. Bach's Leo moon (21° 25′) appears in the Second House with several challenging aspects. In her book, *The Essence of Bach Flowers,* * astrologer and Registered Bach Practitioner, Rachelle Hasnas, identifies the Leo moon with Bach's remedy, *Vervain.* On this basis, then, Bach would be assumed to have a Vervain soul-type. However, this could be open to debate as several who knew him personally identified him as an Impatiens soul. Barnard observes that there is a fine distinction in diagnosis between the Impatiens and Vervain characteristics. He points out that Vervain is mental, while Impatiens works on a 'feeling' response.† Certainly, we can ascribe both characteristics to Bach's soul-type. However, for a brief moment, it is interesting to simply to focus on the astrological interpretations according to Bach's own hypothesis.

The moon being part of a fixed T-square with his Taurus Neptune (27°40′) and Scorpio Mars (22°32′), Bach may have been someone who in past lives was used to being in charge and having his own way. However, he probably paid very dearly for this attitude. His natal moon placing would also indicate that he struggled with the conflict between material comfort and spiritual evolution. In this light, it is interesting to recall that as a young man he *knew* he was to be a healer. The debate within himself was whether to follow this path through medicine or the ministry. While he initially chose the path of potential material comfort through medicine, it was not long before he began to feel the binding confines of traditional medicine. This discomfort, or conflict with his soul's intent, could be the driving factor

*1999, The Crossing Press, Freedom, California.   †Barnard 2002

behind his decision to disconnect from the way medicine was practised, but not from the business of healing.

The moon, which symbolizes our feminine aspect and feelings, is the ruling planet in Bach's chart. If we consider Bach's personal philosophy stating that there is a relationship between astrological moon signs and the Twelve Healers, this presents us with additional intriguing considerations. Unfortunately, we do not have Bach's personal scheme of the specific links between the zodiacal moon signs, the Twelve Healers, and their soul lessons. However, if we consider Bach as Vervain soul-type according to the scheme proposed by Hasnas and other astrologers familiar with the characteristics of the remedies and soul types, we have to consider the characteristics of Vervain according to Bach's own observations. Among them are possession of high ideals and 'ambitions for the good of humanity'.* There is also an aspect to Vervain that desires to 'right all wrongs'; the problem with these desires is when the 'enthusiasm' of the Vervain soul converts into a state of zealousness. Nevertheless, as a Vervain soul, Bach would have been very concerned with doing all he could in correcting conditions he viewed as unjust. This personal perception would have extended to his desire to aid or support individuals whom he deemed as being unfairly treated in life. This then, along with his Cancer ascendant (28° 50´) supports his personal path of reflecting upon all aspects of the human condition and to act upon his conclusions. Fortunately, for us, Bach was wise enough to listen to the voice of his soul, his intuition.

At some point, however, Bach apparently became concerned that those who had no interest in or were not sympathetic to astrological philosophy would disregard the healing benefits of the remedies. By all indications, to address this concern, he ceased public reference to the relationship between the remedies and astrology. It is doubtful however, being the student of the esoteric that he was, that he dropped his personal interested in the subject. In a letter written in the fall of 1933, Bach states:

> I am being very cautious as regards astrology, and that is why one left out the Signs and the months in the first Twelve Healers. This work is decidedly going to assist vastly in the purification and understanding of astrology, but my part seems to be to give general principles whereby people like you who have a more detailed knowledge, may discover a great truth. That is why I do not wish to be associated with anything dogmatic, until one is sure.*

In any case, he did not abandon his focus on the connection between the Twelve Healers and the lessons of the soul-personality types.

On our own journey, we have the opportunity of discovering that the remedies can speak to us on levels of unimagined connection. If we are able to understand that they are here to increase our soul-awareness as we travel our path, they can take us into realms we never would have imagined, or possibly chosen, for ourselves. On the other hand, if in this incarnation we are not ready for this connection or journey, we need to recall that the spiritual train will not leave without us and that cosmic law dictates that we will have future opportunities.

This then brings us to the point of asking, *what is the story in our soul?*

*Original Writings, p. 87.

CHAPTER SIX

AS ABOVE, SO BELOW: TRANSFORMING SOUL-LESSONS OF HEAVEN AND EARTH

'The most beautiful and most profound emotion we can experience is the sensation of the mystical. It is the source of all true science. He to who the emotion is a stranger, who can no longer wonder and stand rapt in awe, is as good as dead'.

ALBERT EINSTEIN

SEVERAL years ago, the neuroscientist, Candace Pert, Ph.D., gave an interview in which she stated: *'Emotions are in two realms. They're in the realm of the physical, the molecular, the material, and they're also in the realm of the spiritual. It's almost like [they are] the transition element.... That's why they are so critically important'.** Coming as it does from a scientist who operates in the world of matter and hard science, this perspective on emotions is profound. It is so because it recognizes that, indeed, our emotions and feelings function not only in the physical realm, but also in a realm that often eludes rational understanding. For this reason, it is vital for each of us that we comprehend we are spirit in body; that we are compelled to walk our path in

Alternative Therapies, July 1995 1:3, p. 73

the temporal realm in order to manifest our soul's fire and vision.

On this journey, our ego can become demanding and hold unrealistic expectations. As a result, when our expectations do not manifest, contracted feelings of anger, greed, bitterness, resentment, fear and a host of other toxic emotions emerge which keep us from soul-growth. Unrealistic expectations that feed these emotions have no place in the realm of the higher mind. On our path, we need to remember that our higher mind is a link with the pure wisdom of our soul through our heart-based intuition. By facilitating a release of the ego's unrealistic expectations, Bach's remedies move us forward toward the growth that the universe intends for each of us.

This release is crucial if we are to move into the Aquarian consciousness of global unity. Furthermore, Bach's concept of the twelve soul-types (or soul-personalities) and their corresponding lessons becomes a significant consideration in the pursuit of discovering our soul-path. In Bach's mind, our soul-type is our core foundation, much like the operating system of computers. As each of us comes into this life with our particular type, we also carry a soul-lesson for us to strengthen (as we saw in the previous chapter). Thus, when we incarnate in this lifetime, our soul-type is in some degree of 'contraction' or weakness with a mandate to work toward 'expansion' or strength through its soul-type lesson.

While we may manifest bits and pieces of various soul-types as we evolve through an incarnation, Bach maintained that, ultimately, each of us remains bonded to one distinct type represented by one of the Twelve Healers. Our soul-type is, in fact, our core foundation in each lifetime.* From a spiritual perspective, it appears that Bach felt that through successive reincarnations we work our way through each of the twelve types and their lessons, similar to the philosophy found in astrology. By strengthening the qualities of the types through their lesson in each life, the soul gleans experience and knowledge and thus moves closer to God.

As Bach's work evolved, an additional twenty-six remedies became part of the repertoire. The work on these was done between 1933 and 1935, at which point he announced his work complete. Since Bach's death in 1936, there have been those who have proposed that several of the additional twenty-six are also 'soul-type' remedies. However, Bach never mentions any of these additional remedies in the context of 'soul-type' remedies; and so it would appear that in his mind, they were not. Thus, from the *spiritual* perspective, it is important to remember that Bach's belief was that the first set of remedies, the Twelve Healers, was there to assist the corresponding soul-types in the transformation of their karmic lessons.

However, we now need to turn from spiritual matters to an examination of the Twelve Healers, the additional twenty-six remedies and their relationship to the healing process on the mundane level. On this level, the Twelve Healers and the twenty-six additional remedies function in a similar way to the concept of 'root and branch herbs' used in oriental medicine or 'constitutional and lower potency' remedies used in homeopathy. In these medical traditions (and in Edward Bach's philosophy), there is always an underlying 'root' cause

*Barnard 2002, p. 283.

for a chronic imbalance, but this cause is not always in evidence. In Chinese medicine, the particular herb (or herbs) used to address the root imbalance is considered the 'principal herb'; and in homeopathy, practitioners look to identify the 'constitutional type' of the patient and its corresponding remedy. However, before these solutions become clearly evident, other support-herbs or homeopathic remedies of various potencies may be needed to assist in balancing out the overlaying symptoms first. Thus, by the clearing away of these symptoms, the imbalance at the 'root of the matter' can then be recognized and addressed. In practice, Bach practitioners refer to this process as a 'peeling of the onion'. If one reads Bach's own words carefully in *The Twelve Healers and Four Helpers,* published by C. W. Daniel Co. in 1933, he clearly lays out his philosophy on this issue as it relates to this concept with the flower remedies:

> *It will be found that certain cases do not seem to fit exactly any one of the Twelve Healers, and many of these are such as those who have become so used to disease that it appears to be part of their nature; and it is difficult to see their true selves because, instead of seeking a cure, they have adapted themselves and altered their lives to suit the disease.... Such people have lost much of their individuality, of their personality, and need to be helped out of the rut, out of the grove, in which they have become fixed before it is possible to know which of the twelve healers they need ... and the Four Helpers get us over this stage and bring us into the range of the Twelve Healers. Of course, in all healing there must be a desire in the patient to get well.* *

Therefore, while it may seem that some of the additional remedies discovered after the Twelve Healers might also be identified as 'soul-types', this appears not to be the case. In-

---

*Barnard, *Collected Writings,* p. 70.

stead, as Bach stressed, there can be emotional issues that
are chronic in nature, so much so that the individual is emotionally 'stuck'. In these circumstances, the remedy or remedies called for may *appear* as soul-type remedies, but the
reality is that while the Twelve Healers can be applied to
temporary or chronic emotional states, the remaining
twenty-six are not meant to be identified as soul-types.

On our journey, we shall need to call upon several of the
additional twenty-six remedies; but in doing so, it is important that we maintain our efforts toward the identification
of our soul-type. Although we may not be able to identify
with certainty our soul-type, there still is great value in this
effort. In it rests the understanding of the obstacles that may
keep us from moving forward both spiritually and tempo-
rally. With the help of the Twelve Healers this, then, is our
starting point: a place from which we can steadily work to
develop the characteristics of our soul's strength. Working
with intent, we can thus move forward on our mystical path.
In addition to the complex patterns of emotions and feelings, each of Bach's twelve soul-types exhibits metaphorical
characteristics of the four elements of nature; earth, air,
water and fire. As was mentioned in earlier chapters, the
purpose found in the spiritual law of reincarnation is to give
the soul opportunity for growth toward perfection through
the vehicle of the body and its emotions. This perpetual journey is often referred to in spiritual teachings as the 'baptism
of the four elements'. Thus, with each incarnation, our soul
has the opportunity of growing more mature through the
lessons of its type in each lifetime. In addition, these teachings also inform us that steady growth does not always

happen in each incarnation. Therefore, there are lifetimes in which we can remain stagnantly attached to our weaknesses or failings. When this happens, we are either too earthbound, ungrounded, floundering or on fire. These emotional states can be so intense or entrenched that we have little chance of connecting to our mystical path or *finding the story in our soul.*

The question then becomes how do we identify our soul-type? While it is not impossible to identify, there is no quick solution, simply because by nature we are challenged to take an objective inventory of our behaviour or ourselves. However, we do have clues at our disposal from both our external and internal environments if we pay attention. These clues, however, can come cloaked in a myriad of configurations.

Psychological theory suggests that we are mirrors for each other. Thus, habits and behaviours of others that we find offensive may in fact be characteristics of our own nature, signalling that we need to take a closer look at ourselves. Other clues may reside in difficult relationships and/or careers that we have consciously but misguidedly chosen. Chronic physical illnesses or accidents also give us a chance to examine ourselves in depth. Such clues that head the pack of likely suspects inform us that habits and/or responses that have been familiar, are now no longer viable if we wish to progress on our path.

So once again our process and progress depends upon our willingness to examine what it is within us that keeps us 'stuck' by recreating the same script over and over, but with different casts of characters. Once we are able to make our list of possibilities for change, we are then able to begin surveying the characteristics of the Twelve Healers not only as remedies to call upon, but as soul-types so that we may get on with our work.

Recalling Bach's philosophy relating to the healing action of the remedies, it is important to remember that it is the positive energy or life-force of each remedy that shifts the contracted characteristics of the particular soul-type into the brilliance of its intended expansion. It is here then, from the spiritual perspective, that we have the opportunity to meet the core of the Twelve Healers and the light that they bring into the obscured aspects of our soul.

The contracted state of the soul-type *Mimulus* is about *fear*, but it is those fears that have earthbound or worldly characteristics. Fear of the dark, fear of flying, fear of mice … indeed things that are of this world and have a name. As a soul-type, the contracted state of Mimulus manifests as visceral fear felt within the very core of the individual and, as an unbridled feeling, it is emotionally toxic. Bach described Mimulus soul-types as being quietly afraid of things that they can name and of things that might never happen. From this perspective, Mimulus types are always 'on guard' against what in the extreme is *anything and everything that has a worldly name.*

The *remedy, Mimulus,* engages the intellect to overcome these fears and the ability to sort through them in a rational fashion that then gives the ability to stand firm in the face of challenges. With the help of this remedy, Mimulus types can work toward their soul-mission, which is to teach the virtue or quality of *sympathy* for others because they can well understand their quiet desperation.

While contracted states of feeling can lead us to become self-absorbed, we can also fluctuate the other way and become what psychologists often label as being co-dependent. Co-dependency is a personality characteristic where the contracted state of the *Centaury* soul lives. With a misaligned earthly passion and desire to serve, Centaury's hindrance or *weakness* is the inability or lack of will to set boundaries by saying: 'No'.

As a result, these individuals become the common doormat by default, doing too much for others while sacrificing their own wellbeing from a severely-skewed altruistic perspective. As with all contracted states of feeling, this particular perspective comes with its own set of difficulties. Foremost among these difficulties is that these individuals unknowingly engineer their own fate as both physical and emotional sacrificial lambs. With the inability to set their own boundaries against the demands of others, they continually 'do' for those around them while their own physical and emotional resources slowly go down the drain. Through their lack of will, it is only when they are 'on the ropes' that they may begin to wonder, if at all, how they arrived at such a state.

Another difficulty with the contracted Centaury soul is that of the well-intended but misguided desire in their attempt to 'fix' problems that others are experiencing. Within the law of karma, our soul sets up difficult relationships and/ or situations meant to offer us opportunities for paying back karmic debt in return for soul-growth. However, when we interfere with others' affairs by attempting to fix their problems, this effort actually stalls *their* soul-path process. As a result, the motivational experience of distress that is required for another's transformation is delayed or altogether derailed.

Here again, we see the inability to set personal boundaries as a major challenge to this aspect of Centaury. Those who incarnate with a Centaury soul and its lesson are natural servers, but the lack of balance creates the inability to stay focused on 'their side of the street'. This behaviour delays their own soul-growth because they are unable to shift towards the expanded state or virtue of *strength of will*. Edward Bach believed that when Centaury types have learned their soul-lesson, with the help of the Centaury remedy, they will have come 'a very long way along the road to being of great service once [they have realized] that [they] must be a little more positive in [their] live[s]'.*

For most of us, the experience of self-doubt and its companion, the feeling of failure, are natural emotions that are part and parcel of the human incarnation. For *Gentian* soul-types however, *self-doubt* is its destructive weakness. In the contracted soul-state, these individuals begin with a positive passion for their direction in life and the tasks that are required to reach their goals. However, when difficulty emerges at the first bend in the road, when an obstacle, no matter how minor appears, discouragement and self-doubt readily take hold. At this juncture, Gentian soul-types who have not progressed in mastering the expanded emotional state of this remedy become easily discouraged, ready to throw in the towel and give up. Recalling Bach's philosophy on failure from the previous chapter, his message was specifically directed to the *Gentian* soul-types *[with the] understanding that there is no failure when you are doing your utmost, whatever the apparent result'.* †

The challenge then for Gentian souls is to embrace the virtue of *understanding*. In order to connect to its soul's fire

*Barnard, 2002, p. 112. †Barnard, *Collected Writings*, p. 107.

and mystical path, the Gentian soul needs to understand that steady perseverance is essential to overcoming self-doubt. While faith in self is important for each of the soul-types, it is particularly important for these individuals. For them, a vital key is to remember that cosmic law dictates trusting the perfect timing of the universe; that the universe provides them with whatever they need for their expansion and growth. For the soul-type who finds change and challenge difficult, Gentian helps them to understand the value of, and engage in, perseverance in the face of adversity and disappointment.

Listening to the wisdom and truth of its own heart and being able to *speak* it is the challenge for a *Cerato* soul. The irony of this soul-type is that it is highly intuitive, but due to the weakness of the contracted state it dwells in *ignorance* or *foolishness,* unable to recognize that its strength is in its own *wisdom.* Lacking in the ability to find its voice, these soul-types have not a clue as to who they are or what they need to do. The weak Cerato soul is not so much one who experiences stolen identity, but one with a case of *lost* identity. Having no faith in its own judgment, the Cerato soul-type perceives its intuitive soul-voice as something that is suspect. Chronically seeking direction from others, they have great difficulty in accessing their higher self and its wisdom and thus have great trouble in finding their intended soul-path.

There is another aspect to Cerato souls. They always want to do the right thing. In this desire, they feed upon the misguided notion that the more information they have, the better off they are in their quest. Unfortunately, this chronic 'gathering' of information from others does nothing other than result in stagnation. Because the contracted Cerato soul is unable to hear, much less listen to its intuitive wisdom in all of its 'gathering', it is never able to act upon anything with conviction. It vacillates, making foolish decisions and taking foolish actions that do nothing but further detain it in its progress. Unable to hold onto a decision, its dependence upon guidance from others creates an appearance of being ungrounded and 'ignorant', one of the very words Bach used to describe the failing of Cerato subjects.

In *Heal Thyself,* Bach notes that, when ill, Cerato types 'try any and every cure suggested'.* It may be that it is the unrealized Cerato types who, in their desperation to learn and do the right thing, lead the pack of the 'sacred shoppers' who fear the spiritual train will leave without them. In working with the *Cerato* remedy, Bach maintained that this soul-type could be 'freed from outside influences, [enabling them] to use the great gift of wisdom that [they] possess for the good of mankind.'§ However, for the contracted Cerato soul, the quality of trusting its intuitive voice and speaking it to guide others lies dormant. They function in the world as a follower, deaf to its intended virtue of wisdom and soul's fire.

Another soul-type that in its contracted state struggles with making decisions is the *Scleranthus* type. However, unlike the Cerato soul who has an identity crisis, Scleranthus types know who they are, but all things being equal, can not decide whether they should wear the black dress or the white dress to the ball, buy the Mini Cooper or the Bentley. While the Cerato soul runs around asking everyone what they

---

*Barnard, *Collected Writings*, p. 84.   †*Collected Writings*, p. 222.   §*Collected Writings*, p. 108.

should do, the Scleranthus soul relies on its intellect while considering its choices. As a result, this individual directs all of its energy to the head and thus cannot verbalize easily. Being unable to have their cake and eat it too results in quiet distress that manifests in first deciding one thing and then another, because all of the options are attractive. Being mental or too much in the head, the contracted Scleranthus soul lacks the ability to access their intuition. Unable to settle on anything requires a tremendous expenditure of energy, draining this individual to the point where they are powerless.

In *Some Fundamental Considerations of Diseases and Cure,* Bach initially called Scleranthus types 'weathervanes', which is an accurate reflection of their inconsistent decision-making skills.* At first glance, such patterns seem identical to those of the contracted Cerato soul. However, in describing the hindrances of the Scleranthus soul, Bach focused on the mental aspect, observing that this type suffers from mental torment. In other words, these soul-types process their dilemmas mentally while the Cerato type has to verbalize its process—two very different ways of being—but neither type can plug into its intuition. Scleranthus' virtue and strength lies in acquiring the ability to remain steadfast in its decisions. Similar to Cerato's soul-issue in this regard, the challenge for the contracted Scleranthus soul is to find comfort in trusting its intuition and letting it be the guide in the decision-making process. In other words, letting the intuitive heart guide the head, not the other way round, is the key for the Scleranthus type in discovering its soul's fire.

The Water Violet plant, according to Barnard, is a very

*Barnard, *Collected Writings,* p. 168.

old one with a complex history that has its mirror in the characteristics of the *Water Violet* soul-type.* In spiritual teachings, those who are considered 'old souls' come into this incarnation possessing a vast storehouse of experience and wisdom; these are the fruits of their labours through many lifetimes. However, the hindrance of the Water-Violet soul is that its history, both karmic and present, has produced a state of *grief*. As is true for each of us, the cosmic laws of karma and rebirth give us the experience of both joy and sorrow. However, for the water-violet soul, a facet of their sorrow or *grief* stems from repeated experiences of betrayal. In their silent grief, the contracted Water Violet comes off as keeping 'a stiff upper lip', while appearing detached, prideful, and aloof. The reality is that this behaviour is a means of emotional protection. Even in simple friendship, intimacy is a hardship for them. Even more of a challenge is finding a level of comfort in the intimacy of a romantic relationship. Physically, the contracted emotional state of this soul-type makes its subjects appear rigid and apart from others, as they exude an air of superiority and entitlement.

Water-violet souls have the lesson this lifetime of learning the virtue of *joy* by sharing their wisdom of experience through participation in the environment that surrounds them. In working through emotional excavation using Water Violet as a remedy, the resulting connection to their feelings brings awareness that detachment is the source of their grief and, what was once good for them—an old defence mechanism that worked—is no longer good for them. When this happens, the emotional armour begins to disintegrate and they

*Barnard, 2002, p. 123.

skilfully learn to balance the need for personal space and the extension of brotherhood through service.

Esoteric tradition teaches that water is the metaphor for feelings and emotions, but among the Twelve Healers, the three soul-types of *Chicory, Clematis and Rock Rose* particularly reflect the sensitivity to emotions and feelings identified with the element of water.

The *Chicory* soul loves to love; but in its contracted state, this soul can become tenacious, self-absorbed, and controlling. As a plant, Chicory adapts to its surrounding environment, manifesting characteristics of changeability in order to fit the situation. This is perhaps why Bach wrote several different descriptions of the negative Chicory soul-type as the repertoire evolved. He was exceptionally critical of the Chicory soul-state in his early paper, *Some Fundamental Considerations on Disease and Cure,* written in 1930. Here he identified Chicory souls as egotistical, spiteful, revengeful and cruel depending on the situation. He later softened his description settling for the word '*restraint*' in describing this type's weakness. While restraint would seem to be an indication of a soul-lesson rather than its weakness, this is not apparently, what Bach saw.

Instead, Bach identified Chicory's weakness as being through emotional manipulation, *unable to restrain itself.* By instigating feelings of guilt (family is a particularly popular target), the contracted Chicory soul-type can go to extremes by contriving situations in order to keep its targets close. Through their manipulations, they succeed in their goal of getting their own way. In many respects, the immature Chicory soul is very needy at a deep level, probably because

*Barnard, *Collected Writings,* p. 165.

this soul has experienced similar parenting dynamics during its own history. Of course, as is the case with each of the soul-types, contracted characteristics can manifest in infancy and the Chicory soul-type is no different. Indications of this state in an infant Chicory soul may surface as constant demands to be held and/or nursed. Furthermore, as the infant grows, the Chicory child can show up as an obstreperous little horror. The danger here is that those whom the Chicory soul is attempting to control may eventually rebel in a dramatic way in order to gain their freedom. This is especially true in the case of a parent who manipulates his or her children under the guise of 'knowing what's best for them'.

Bach described the strength of this soul-type as *love*; making the point that we gain love by giving others freedom without expectation. In working with the Chicory remedy, subjects of this soul-type mature on finding that by giving freedom rather than holding on, they gain a far deeper and more global love than they ever thought possible.

Returning just briefly to Bach's thoughts on astrology and the soul-types, we find that according to Hasnas and other astrologers familiar with Bach's work, the Clematis soul is represented by the sign of Cancer, traditionally ruled by the Moon. In other words, you will not find a Clematis personality in someone with a Leo moon. In addition to astrological philosophy that dictates Cancer is ruled by the moon rather than one of the planets, spiritual teachings traditionally connect the moon to the feminine aspect of our energy, our spiritual heart. Symbolically the moon, because it reflects the light of the sun, which is the representation of our masculine energy, represents all our emotions, feelings, and intuitive self.

Cultures around the world depict the lunar magic of the moon through myths, fairy tales, and stories. 'By the light of the moon', 'dreaming in the light of the moon', 'mooning over someone' in romantic ardour all relate to emotional states with a dreamlike quality. Thus, it is not so surprising that the weakness of the Clematis soul is that of *indifference* which shows up by appearing ungrounded and dreamy.

In *Some Fundamental Considerations of Disease and Cure,* Bach originally described the Clematis soul as 'the ecstatic'.* If we can recall from Chapter Four that we are all 'called to be mystics', we may appreciate that characteristics of ecstasy such as 'bliss or 'rapture' that have been identified with some 'mystics', are not necessarily a prerequisite for mysticism. In other words, not all mystics are ecstatics or Clematis souls. However, when identifying the 'hindrance state' of the Clematis soul-type, Bach was referring to those souls who chronically prefer to escape into the realms of their ideals and visions with little concern for or fear of, illness or death. As a defence mechanism, and to protect their highly-sensitive natures, these individuals, like the crab, retreat into their shell when faced with problems or difficult realities. For the contracted Clematis soul, living in the reality of the present seems too harsh and overwhelming; it is as if they cannot muster the internal strength to interact with even the very ordinary details of life. Thus, their heightened sensitivity to the energy and emotional states of others and their own surrounding environment makes this method of escape their modus operandi; they simply are not present. This state of non-presence can manifest in a varied assortment of both

*Barnard, *Collected Writings*, p. 165.

physical and mental behaviours. Contracted states of the Clematis soul can range from daydreaming, fainting, or Attention Deficit Disorder to the extreme of dementia or Alzheimer's disease.

The virtue or strength of the Clematis soul is one of *gentleness*, but it is a virtue that can only be realized with stability and a sense of being grounded into the earth through its soul-remedy. The Clematis remedy assists these souls in becoming earthbound so that they may respond self-assuredly with gentleness, rather than retreating in escape. With their sensitivity to others and the world around them, Clematis soul-types have the opportunity and responsibility to teach the rest of the world the value of extending gentleness to each other … a virtue that is sorely needed in today's world and an absolute necessity for spreading global brotherhood.

As with all of the water signs in astrology, heightened sensitivity is an issue with a two-edged sword. For the *Rock Rose* soul, this sensitivity is more heightened than we find in either Chicory or Clematis souls. At the cellular level, for the Rock Rose soul-type there is an awareness of vulnerability that conveys a palpable terror. Just the 'business of being' is terrifying; and thus *terror* is the weakness or hindrance for these souls. For them, this weakness manifests in a constant emotional undercurrent of belief about 'not coming through it', whatever 'it' is. Interestingly, this undercurrent can remain well-hidden until that time when it bursts up and out, manifesting into a full-blown, paralysing panic attack. Unlike the visible timidity and nervousness of the Mimulus soul, the hidden terror of the Rock Rose soul is really only recognizable to those of like soulfulness. In other words, 'it takes one to know one'. It is very difficult for the non-Rock Rose soul to detect this in others because of this remarkable ability of the Rock Rose to 'stuff it'. In reality, the accurate identification of a Rock Rose soul-type only becomes a conscious consideration when the contracted characteristics visibly manifest in chronic episodes of panic and terror.

From a karmic perspective, the contracted soul-state of Rock Rose is not something that has just come about in this lifetime. More than likely, this state of contraction is a result of many lifetimes in which they have experienced the 'fires of hell', so to speak, and consequently paralysing terror has become a thematic state of being. Bach identified these souls as being terrified of things other than the material, such as death, suicide, or the supernatural. Thus, according to Bach, with the help of its soul-remedy, the lesson or positive quality for the Rock Rose soul to develop in this lifetime is *courage*. As these souls learn to become comfortable with the emotional state of courage, they begin to expand and are progressively able to stand firm in their place. By standing with courage, they are further able to *displace* the contracted emotional shadow of terror that has made their lives difficult and fraught with unrealized contributions to humanity. By coming to grips with this debilitating emotion, they are then in a position to teach others that, we are divinely protected and therefore, terror *is only a shadow*.

Having explored the metaphors of the emotions of the earth, air, and water, we now come to the nature of the emotions of the last element, those of fire.

Seemingly the ever-present diplomat, avoiding all confrontation, the *Agrimony* soul appears as the peacemaker who is very much 'out there' with boundless energy actively connected in and to the world. There is only one small problem … what the rest of the world is seeing is the contracted Agrimony soul-type, and as such, it is the master of disguise. The contracted Agrimony soul fools the world. This type appears to others as *the one* who 'has it together' but the reality is that its weakness is its *restlessness* at the soul level. Behind every smile, every laugh, this contracted soul-type struggles with its restlessness in quiet torment that no-one else ever sees. It simply cannot find the *peace* that is its lesson and strength. Without question, the worst thing for a contracted Agrimony soul is that its secret torment will be revealed and that it will be found out. In order to cope, contracted Agrimony will hide, often unconsciously, its torment by retreating to the use of drugs, alcohol, or other addictive behaviours. This method of retreat or 'protection' of course only creates more difficulties.

It is almost as if the contracted Agrimony soul is in the wrong incarnation, the wrong body, and thus trying unsuccessfully to throw it off, like too many covers on the bed. The reality is that from the spiritual perspective, they are in the right body, the right place at the right time. The challenge for the contracted Agrimony soul is to become comfortable with revealing who and particularly *how* they really are. In the contracted state, these souls will reply that they are 'just fine' when asked; never mind that they have just filed bankruptcy, their partner has left them, and that government revenue agents have them on their 'most-wanted list' for tax misunderstandings. Agrimony as a remedy assists these souls in developing the ability to be verbally honest about their state of being. Once they begin to work with this challenge, they find that their restlessness dissipates and in their liberation, they can move forward on their mystical path through their soulful quality of *peace*. In writing about the lesson of peace for Agrimony, Bach said:

> *Does not Agrimony 'open the door to let in the golden vital breath of peace instead of love. One always feels that the light of Agrimony is so very closely associated with 'the peace that passeth understanding', the peace of the Christ;*

Although peace is the specific soul-lesson for Agrimony, Bach also made it a repetitive theme, woven in throughout his philosophy. In his address, *Ye Suffer From Yourselves,* he identifies the state of peace as being one of the basic components required for healing. Bach 'saw' that a hospital of the future would be:

> *a sanctuary of peace, hope and joy. No hurry; no noise: entirely devoid of all the terrifying apparatus and appliances of today.... The object of all institutions will be to have an atmosphere of peace, and of hope, of joy, and of faith.*

If you are launching a new enterprise that requires collective participation, particularly an effort that focuses upon fighting for justice, get an 'expanded' *Vervain* soul on your steering committee—if you can find one. More than likely, however, you will be confronted by the over-zealous enthusiasm of a contracted Vervain soul who is on a mission. In this state, these soul-types can be extremely difficult to work with. Unlike contracted Agrimony, who struggles with his or her personal experience of microcosm versus macrocosm, contracted Vervain simply is dissatisfied with the entire macrocosmic set-up. In the contracted extreme, the Vervain souls are frothing at the mouth, determined. They will to

do everything possible to get their oar into the water, pad-
dling furiously to engineer the tides of change—for the bet-
terment of humankind, of course, or their next-door
neighbour.

Among the Twelve Healers, Bach identified Vervain as the
'enthusiast'. In its contracted state, the Vervain soul suffers
from an over-abundance of a driving force whose weakness
or hindrance is one of *over-enthusiasm*. Emotional fire of this
nature translates into intolerance of others and ideas that
do not match Vervain's own. Because these souls have travelled far on their journey, they have developed an indomi-
table spirit and bring with them very clear ideals of 'how
things should be'. The problem is not in the intent, but in
the application; the contracted Vervain soul hits the ground
running, taking no prisoners.

Those whom we experience in this way may or may not
be actual Vervain types. However, if they are, it is quite possible that they have karmically chosen to be in relationships
that exhibit similar behaviour either through demand for
high achievement, critical role-models, or both. This being
the case, the contracted Vervain soul has the option of remaining stagnant by mimicking these behaviours and philosophies or embracing its soul-remedy to assist it as it learns
the lesson of *tolerance*. Bach identified Vervain's potential
power as that seen in leaders and effective teachers. Should
contracted Vervain souls take the option of learning tolerance, they can embrace this power through the spiritual
axiom that all great work can be accomplished quietly.

While poor contracted Centaury struggles to learn about
setting boundaries, the fiery *Impatiens* soul knows exactly

where the boundaries are and wants to burn them down; the sooner, the better. In its very nature, the contracted Impatiens soul is a bundle of combustible energy in thought and action. This type is blessed with a quicksilver mind, but when it gets entrenched in its failing of *impatience*, it perceives everything and everyone around it as unnecessary and irrelevant restrictions.

In other words, 'get out of my way' is its message to the world and Impatiens manifests this by striking out, through caustic verbiage and visible irritation. If the Impatiens soul does not move forward in learning its lesson of *forgiveness*, it finds that it has alienated those around it and is destined to lead a lifetime of loneliness. In the process of learning its lesson of forgiveness, the Impatiens souls are challenged to recognize that not everyone thinks like, or as fast, as they do. A major key to attaining progress on their mystical path is by working with their soul-remedy, Impatiens. This remedy assists the Impatiens soul in becoming aware that others have gifts to offer and that we are all connected through our contributions and universal brotherhood.

As with each of the soul-types, it is impossible for us to know why one individual comes into this incarnation with a particular soul-lesson to learn in lieu of another. Barnard and others confidently identify Bach as an Impatiens type,* given his penchant for working alone, his quickness of mind and vacillating behaviour. Interestingly, if we return to the astrological concept of the natal moon as a key to identifying one's soul-type, then Bach with his Leo moon would be identified as a Vervain soul, as we saw. It is interesting to note

*Barnard, 2002, p. 32.

that in sketching a verbal profile of Bach, his close colleague, Dr. F. J. Wheeler, notes that:

His intense desire to help others to understand and learn as quickly as he did himself sometimes made him impatient at slowness, but this mood would not last long [author note: Impatiens characteristics] . . . although he was quick to anger at injustice, unhesitatingly voicing it and siding with the weaker [author note: Vervain characteristics], he would encourage the weak one to fight his own battles and so regain his self-esteem.

It may be that Bach himself was an example of one of those individuals whose overlaying characteristics are so strong that it is tricky to identify the soul-type. Thus, perhaps to the world Bach appeared as an Impatiens type when actually he was a Vervain soul, clearly on a karmic mission for this lifetime. Bach may have been one of those people with whom the personality characteristics (Impatiens) were so entrenched that they hid the actual soul-type (Vervain). As I indicated earlier, uncertainty of the astrological scheme was the reason that Bach dropped *public* mention of connection between the remedies and astrology. Then again, the possibility of obtaining clarity in this matter with certainty is maybe one that will be denied us. What is paramount to remember, however, is that the remedies can bring unique awareness, lessons, and experience to each of us in our efforts to identify and work our intended soul-lesson for this lifetime. As healing tools, *The Twelve Healers* can meet us where we are; and if we are willing to follow, they can take us where our soul wants us to be.

CHAPTER SEVEN

THE SEVEN SACRED GATES OF SOUL-AWARENESS: THE CHAKRAS*

It has been said that the eyes are the windows to the soul. But in some spiritual teachings and ancient mystery schools the chakras are considered gateways, or portals, to our soul's wisdom.

AMONG THE many aspects of Bach's thought that appear throughout his writings are those that bring his spiritual nature to light. Through his writings he informs us that in conjunction with the remedies themselves, he had a symbiotic relationship with all things that he considered divinely inspired, including philosophies of the East. On more than one occasion, in reference to a variety of subjects, Bach refers to the teachings of 'the Lord Buddha', 'Our Mother India', and other 'Masters'. He places these references within the context of their importance to healing in that how we live, and the spiritual process used to do so, helps us to discover our soul's fire, and therefore, our soul-agenda:

We have the glorious example, the great standard of perfection and the teachings of The Christ to guide us. . . . His mission on earth was to teach us how to

*Portions of this chapter were originally published in *The International Journal of the Sacred Space Foundation*, Fall quarter, 2003.

*obtain harmony and communication with our Higher Self. . . . Thus also taught
the Lord Buddha and other great Masters, who have come down from time to
time upon earth to point out to men the way to attain perfection. . . .*★

Although absolute evidence does not seem to be available,
it is reasonable to presume that among the various facets of
these philosophies Bach developed a working knowledge of
the 'chakras'.

The identification of the chakras is anchored in the ancient yogic tradition of Hinduism and, later, Buddhism. We
may find through our sacred shopping a plethora of authori-
tative works on the subject of the chakras: what they are,
what they do and how they affect us. As always in discus-
sions of spiritual beliefs, there are subtle variances in philosophy. No less is true when one considers the chakras and
their relationship to 'auras'. In esoteric traditions, it is generally accepted that there is an 'envelope' of vital energy that
radiates from everything in nature, including the human
body, known as an aura. To clairvoyants, auras manifest as
energetic layers of colours. These layers surrounding the
body continuously expand and contract in the intensity of
their colours and in their boundaries. Interestingly, the concept of auras and energy actually dates back to the ancient
world appearing 'in the writings and art of Egypt, India,
Greece, and Rome where saints appear wreathed with ha-
loes. In the sixteenth century, Paracelsus was one of the first
western scholars to expound upon the astral body, which
he described as a fiery globe'.†

Fundamental to the concept of chakras is that they are

★Barnard, *Collected Writings*, p. 156. †*Harper's Encyclopedia of Mystical and Paranormal Experience*, p 40.

seven major centres (in addition to hundreds of minor ones)
that continually vibrate as they process the energy within
the various layers of our 'aura'. These seven chakras function in each of our auric layers, i.e., the etheric, astral, and
mental bodies. In addition, they have a relationship to our
physical body through the pathways of our central nervous
system that lie along our spinal column.

When we move into emotional states of distress, consciously or unconsciously, the negative energy of our emotions initiates patterns of contraction within the chakras and
our auras. Like the pebble tossed into a pond of still water,
this action perpetuates disruptive permutations that reverberate throughout these layers. Spiritual writings and philosophy of the East teach that the ultimate result of block-
ages to positive energetic flow manifests in illness and disease.
Conversely, when we experience positive emotional states,
the chakras intensify and expand into harmonic balance.

As spirit in body, our soul is constantly pushing us toward this harmony within and amongst these centres, with
the goal of bringing them into full expansion and expression for our highest good. This process of soul-growth is one
that leads us through the delicate intricacies of emotional
balance between needing connection and courage, choice
and resilience, self-love and unconditional love, emotional
voice and authority, and insight and faith. Thus, working
with these images, we find that the emotional imprints of
the chakras are excellent maps for discovering unexplored
territory. In this way, the nature of emotions both positive
and negative is cellular fuel. The energy or vibrations of nega-

*Harper's Encyclopedia of Mystical and Paranormal Experience, p 86.

tive emotional imprints within the chakras not only facilitate a contraction from soul-connection but, conversely, positive emotional imprints facilitate expansion toward the soul. Moreover, this process is as fluid as mercury.

It follows, then, that when our emotions shut down, or we are emotionally 'stuck', the vibration within the chakras enters into a state of contraction, thereby resulting in operational shaky ground or no foundation at all. In order to bring our chakras into states of expansion, our emotional excavation needs to begin by exploring *where* we become emotionally stuck and *why*. Further, and most importantly, *what* tools do we have at our disposal that can assist us in our endeavours to move out of our toxic spaces? It is here that we can look at the emotional imprints of the seven chakras and their relationship to the Bach remedies.

Recalling that the core of Bach's philosophy on the nature of healing focused on the relationship between polar opposites, the connection between the positive energy of the remedies and contracted or negative states of the chakras becomes evident as he states,

> *if a patient has a mental [emotional] error, a conflict between physical and spiritual self will result, and disease will be the product. The error may be repelled, the poison driven from the body, but a vacuum is left, an adverse force has gone, but a space exists where it has been situated.*
>
> *The perfect method is not so much to repel the adverse influence, as to draw in its opposing virtue; and by means of this virtue, flood out the fault. This is the law of opposites, of positive and negative.* *

Taking this perspective a step further, the positive energy or vibrations of the remedies are capable of catalysing subtle

*Barnard, *Collected Writings*, p. 159.

but broad transformations within the numerous and often complex layers of our emotions. Thus, appropriate combinations of the remedies shift as our internal perspectives shift, facilitating an ongoing expansion of our chakras and shifts in our external behaviours.

As we have already seen, Bach had a fascination with numbers and, it appears, with certain numbers in particular. Keeping in mind that there are seven major chakras, this number repeatedly appears in Bach's work. Between 1928 and 1930, Bach initially worked out identifying characteristics of seven behavioural groups that he felt were keys to an individual's ability to recover from illness and disease. Within these seven groups, he further identified specific qualities of what he called temporary 'mood states' and the more established 'personality types'. He labelled the inclusive nature of these categories as 'Fear, Uncertainty, Insufficient Interest in Present Circumstances, Loneliness, Over-Sensitivity to Influences and Ideas, Despondency and Despair, and Over-concern for Welfare of Others'.*

As the work with the remedies progressed over the years, Bach continued to fine-tune this aspect of his work, including the placement of each of the thirty-eight remedies into one of the seven categories. This approach emphasized the heart of his insights on the actual *treatment* of illness and disease. His belief was that when faced with illness, each of us reacts emotionally according to our 'group' mood state or personality type. We do *not* react according to the symptoms of the particular illness or disease. Here again, at the heart of this theory, we find the number 'seven'.*

*Weeks, *Discoveries*, pp. 39–40.

Barnard observes that in all likelihood Bach's working knowledge of the seven-chakra system corresponded to the headings for his mood/personality groups. The number of these groups, however, was not the only parallel. Bach concluded that there were also 'seven principles' in which a personality may err in its soul-evolution, a conclusion which he presented in *Some Fundamental Considerations of Disease and Cure* (published in 1930). In this work, Bach identifies these as 'power, intellectual knowledge, love, balance, service, wisdom and spiritual perfection.'.† He later altered his 'seven principles' into 'the 'seven' beautiful stages of healing: 'love, wisdom, certainty, faith, joy, hope and peace'.§

As noted earlier, Bach intended his system of healing to be one of simplicity; but certainly there is contradiction between this desire and the nature of Bach, himself. In reading what little is available of his own writings, it is evident that he was constantly fine-tuning his theories of application, while remaining steadfast in his approach to all things spiritual. As such, his methodology and thought-processes are sometimes confusing and sometimes too intellectual.

Thus, when he was speaking of mood-states and personality-types in context of his seven groups, he was addressing issues of methodology for treating illness. He did not intend that this approach to treating illness be confused with his earlier writings on soul-lessons and the karmic law of rebirth in reference to the Twelve Healers as soul-types. Thus, re-emphasizing a point I made earlier, he worked simultaneously on both the mundane and spiritual planes

---

*Barnard, *Collected Writings*, pp. 35–36. †Barnard, 2002 p. 281. §Barnard, *Collected Writings*, p. 101.

with his remedies. It is not always easy to be certain of Bach's internal thought-processes or which 'personal lens' he was looking through. In this regard, such confusion on our part seems to be more about his desire constantly to learn and expand upon what he already knew or was 'shown' (a distinction we noted in earlier chapters), rather than not being sure of his knowledge. Despite the constant amendments to his observations of human nature, it seems that in his mind, there were connections between the traditional characteristics of each major chakra, personality, or mood-types, and stages of healing.

In 1934, when Bach settled at Mt Vernon for the last two years of his life, he had thus far identified the twelve soul-types, the Twelve Healers, and the Seven Helpers.* Although he believed his work was now complete, this was not to be. During 1935, he discovered what we know today as the final nineteen remedies. These were the remedies that he considered 'more spiritualized', functioning at a higher vibration than the original 'twelve' soul-type remedies or the additional 'seven helpers'.†

The significance of these additional nineteen is that they relate to *emotional responses* that we may have to 'in the moment' events. However, these events, although current, can also fire emotions tied to our personal history through our subconscious memories. Even though we are not conscious of these connections, our subconscious connection to the deep and subtle familiarity of past experiences creates an instant reaction that manifests in the same fears, insecurity,

---

*The seven helpers are Olive, Gorse, Oak, Vine, Heather, Rock Water and Wild Oat. †Barnard, *Collected Writings*, p. 23.

apathy, guilt, or shame. Often such reactions are referred to as 'hot buttons' or 'knee-jerk reactions'. The bad news is that we are so comfortable with these responses that we do not realize that we have a *very unhealthy history with them.*

Since Bach was also a homoeopath, there is a parallel of the spiritual axiom 'as above, so below' in homeopathic theory. Homeopathy is considered vibrational or energy medicine. In terms of potency or the vibration of the homeopathic remedy, the philosophy is that those remedies with higher vibrations heal at deeper levels within us. In Bach's observation, the final nineteen remedies functioned at a 'higher vibration'. In that function, he was also saying that their efficacy was capable of balancing out toxic emotions at very deep levels.

From an energetic perspective, the emotional patterns of our chakras are about as deep as you can excavate—should you wish to go there. More often than not, we try to pass on this, saying to ourselves, *I think I'll negotiate, I'll do anything but THAT; it isn't so bad.* The conflict here is that our soul is trying to push us *into its fire* but as humans, we are internally wired to resist this push initially. While we consciously believe we are 'in charge', our resistance plays out through repetitive history that is toxic. Unaware that our soul's will is far wiser and more powerful, our resistance eventually brings us to our knees either physically or metaphorically—sometimes both. Furthermore, it is at this point, as we teeter on the edge of our personal abyss, that we ask ourselves in wonderment, 'How the blazes did I get here?'

This is the moment when we need to take an inventory of our chakras, their emotional patterns, and our participation in how we 'got here'. Fortunately, we have tools to work with, our twelve soul-types, the seven helpers, and the final nineteen remedies. This is the moment when we take the plunge, board the spiritual train with our karmic and current emotional baggage, and head toward our destination: our soul's fire.

> *[These] beautiful remedies, which have been Divinely enriched with healing powers, . . . open up those channels to limit more light of the Soul, that [we] may be flooded with healing virtue. . . . The action of these remedies is to raise our vibrations and open up our channels for the reception of our Spiritual Self, to flood our natures with the particular virtue we need. . . . They cure, not by attacking disease, but by flooding our bodies with the beautiful vibrations of our Higher Nature, in the presence of which disease melts as snow in the sunshine.* *

*Barnard, *Collected Writings*, p. 117.

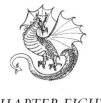

CHAPTER EIGHT

IT'S ALL IN THE CHAKRAS

WHETHER we respond to our environment with faith or fear
depends in large part upon the emotional and energetic patterns rooted in our chakras. These patterns, when expanded,
bring us into a state of authentic balance, wellbeing and faith.
However, because we incarnate into this lifetime with karma
to burn off, our chakra patterns typically fluctuate between
contraction and expansion. As we burn off our karmic debt
this fluctuation cycle is part of the process through which
we heal old emotional wounds and at the same time create
new ones. Unfortunately, one of the difficulties that we encounter in this process is that for most of us it usually takes
a physical malfunction for the problem to get our attention. Western medicine would have us believe that the true
nature of being 'healed' is manifested by the absence of disease. From a spiritual point of view, and certainly from
Edward Bach's perspective, healing goes far deeper than our
physical, cellular, self. True healing is the transformation
not only of body, but also of mind and emotions, down into
the depths of our *spirit*. This is a goal we are compelled to
work toward, one that is fuelled by our soul's intent that we
connect to its purpose through the purification-fires of our
feelings and emotional process.

In the previous chapter, I set out the seven stages of healing that Bach identified: *peace, hope, joy, faith, certainty, wisdom and love,* in that order. But, if we consider these stages in a different order, as they relate to the traditional themes of the seven chakras, a very interesting scenario takes shape. Additionally, if we consider the relationship between the final nineteen remedies (i.e., those identifying emotions 'reactionary' to our environment), the seven steps of healing and the seven chakras, we are presented with an opportunity that can help us to not only progress further along our mystical path, but to discover our soul's fire.

While Bach believed that the final nineteen remedies were more spiritualized and functioned at a higher vibration, it is important to remember that they are no more important than the first nineteen. However, although there are approximately over two hundred million combinations of Dr Bach's thirty-eight remedies,* the final nineteen are particularly valuable tools in our exploration of the emotional patterns lodged in our chakras. While each of the remedies meets us where we are, helping us to get where we need to be, the connection between emotional discord and physical imbalance is a prevailing theme that appears throughout Bach's writings. In *Heal Thyself,* he states:

> *It cannot be too firmly realized that every soul in incarnation is down here for the specific purpose of gaining experience and understanding, and of perfecting his personality towards those ideals laid down by the soul. No matter what our relationship be to each other, whether husband and wife, parent and child, brother and sister, or master and man, we sin against our Creator and against our fellowmen if we hinder from motives of personal desire the evolution of*

*Mathematical source: A. Nelson & Sons, Ltd.

another soul. Our sole duty is to obey the dictates of our own conscience. . . . Let everyone remember that his Soul has laid down for him a particular work, and that unless he does this work, though perhaps not consciously, he will inevitably raise a conflict between his Soul and personality which of necessity reacts in the form of physical disorders. *

In this statement, although it is somewhat lengthy, Bach was very clear about potential outcomes for anyone who chooses to ignore their soul's agenda. For those of us in pursuit of discovering our soul's fire on our mystic path, contraction and imbalance are obstacles to moving forward. Thus, the importance of attaining a sense of emotional wellbeing cannot be overstated. Unfortunately, we are not always able to take an 'objective pulse' of where there are contracted emotional patterns in our chakras. Sometimes we are in such a state of emotional discord that we cannot even see where we are, much less be able to make the connection between the problem and the remedies we need.

Caroline Myss has a favourite expression heard many times by those who attend her workshops and have read her books: 'your biography is your biology'. While this seems a simple statement, the observation is a basic tenet of holistic and integrative medicine. Whatever important discord or distress remains unresolved in your story, your body will eventually manifest it through a physical imbalance of one kind or another; just as was put forward by Dr Bach over seventy years ago.

In exploring the state of the emotional patterns of our chakras, Myss' statement points the way to a very important

*Barnard, *Collected Writings*, p. 140.

map for us. In the true sense of holistic healing, there is never any one solution, as there are many parts to the whole. For example, we can attain a greater sense of self-awareness through our feelings and emotions, but we also can look to physical clues from our body. For some, paying attention to physical clues may be a more obvious pathway to recognizing that there are imbalances in their chakras. The expression, 'listen to your body', is not an idle one. By being able to identify 'where it hurts', we have clues as to where we are stuck through the emotional and physical themes of each of the chakras. Once we are able to identify our 'contracted theme(s)', we can turn to the remedies to assist us in moving from a contracted emotional state to an expansive state, setting us straight on our mystical path.

In two of her books, *Anatomy of the Spirit* (1996) and *Why People Don't Heal and How They Can* (1997) Myss presents both emotional and physical issues that can manifest for each chakra. These are listed in abbreviated format as follows.

Chakra	Organs	Mental/Emotional Issues	Physical Dysfunctions
First	Base of spine immune system	Family & group safety/security	Depression, chronic lower back pain, immune disorders

---

*As I noted in Chapter Seven, there are many credible interpretations of the chakra system. However, for the purposes of this book, I have chosen to use a selection of Myss' interpretations because their transpersonal nature in large part is in line with Dr Bach's philosophy and the healing characteristics of the remedies. A more complete listing of her interpretations can be found in both *Anatomy of Spirit* and *Why People Don't Heal and How They Can*.

Chakra	Organs	Mental/Emotional Issues	Physical Dysfunctions
Second	Sexual organs, regions up to small intestine	Blame, guilt, creativity, power	Chronic lower back pain, sexual difficulties, sciatica
Third	Abdomen, stomach, regions up to the heart	Trust, self-esteem, sensitivity to criticism	Arthritis, colon/ intestinal problems liver dysfunction
Fourth	Heart, lungs, breasts,	Love, hatred, resentment grief, hope	Cardiac/pulmonary difficulties, allergies, breast cancer
Fifth	Throat, teeth hypothala- mus	Personal expression, Addiction	Mouth and throat difficulties
Sixth	Brain/ nervous system	Truth, self- evaluation intelligence	Neurological difficul ties, seizures, learn- ing disabilities
Seventh	Muscular, skeletal systems, skin	Faith, spirituality ability to see larger picture	Energetic disorders, extreme sensitivities to environmental factors

In reviewing Myss' interpretations, we may note that she addresses these relationships in the extreme. Clearly, imbalances in the chakras can and do exist without manifesting to such extremes. Taking these concepts to a much broader and deeper level in the chapters that follow, we will be making a *considered and introspective assessment* of how contracted and expanded emotional patterns within our chakras influence our *mental, physical and spiritual health.* This examination is a necessary part of our personal excavation, because it holds the remedy clues from Dr Bach's Final Nineteen as necessary tools in order for us to discover our soul's fire. In these chapters, we will be encouraged to pay attention to the clues offered us with suggestions for remedy solutions that can aid us in working toward chakra expansion and interconnected harmony.

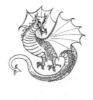

CHAPTER NINE

TAKING ROOT: THE FIRST CHAKRA

Walnut & Cherry Plum—Hope

'The past is never where you think you left it.'
KATHERINE ANNE PORTER

As IN ALL things of an esoteric nature, there are subtle differences in interpretations, but it is generally accepted that the
'physical' locations of our first six chakras are represented
by two triangles, one with a broad base and the point above
and the other the inversion of this, forming the spiritually-
significant, six-pointed star. In this imagery, the Root, Sacral, and Solar plexus chakras exist in the lower triangle. Our
diaphragm (the organ in our body responsible for regulat-
ing our breathing), is the physiological separation between
these chakras with the upper triangle symbolizing the Heart,
Throat and Brow chakras. The crown or seventh chakra is
generally considered non-physical as it is located above the
crown of the head. Thus, some spiritual teachings inform
us that the emotional chakra patterns of the lower triangle
play out through relationships of our physical life, while
those of the upper triangle are more concerned with our

spiritual awakening.* As we continue on our mystical path, however, it is important to keep in mind that the emotional patterns and imprints within *each* chakra influence our relationships. Regardless whether they are in a state of contraction or expansion, the state of our chakras influences our relationships physically, emotionally and spiritually.

According to schools of Eastern philosophical thought, our first chakra is located at the base of the spine. This chakra is where we take root, so to speak; it is in the place which grounds us into the earth. Foundations in general are exceedingly important in our lives, because in form and function they are the underpinnings of the structures and environments in which we live and work. In our body, our feet and legs provide our foundational support for the physical core in which we live. If the foundations that support us in a physical, philosophical, and energetic sense are unstable, we are indeed on very shaky ground.

From both energetic and psychological perspectives, the first chakra is where we connect to our tribe or family identity. This chakra is also the reference and anchor of our mettle and our mission in this life. In the grander scheme of things, when this chakra is in an expanded state, we are acutely aware of the Divine Universe and our connection to it. Unfortunately, achieving this connection is not easy. Nevertheless, we continue to pursue our sacred shopping in order to do so. Universal connection and brotherhood are the goal of the expansion of our first chakra. Our job is to work toward that goal.

Conversely, the first chakra is where our belief-systems are

*Hodgson, *Stars and Chakras*, p. 75.

challenged. Such challenges bring us face to face with an assortment of conflicts manifesting in emotional chaos and physical difficulties. How does this happen? It happens by plugging into a family or tribal agenda that superficially feels appropriate to us. The reality is that this agenda can be, and often is, in conflict with our soul's agenda. The repetitive message in Bach's philosophy, that each of us has a soul-job to do in this life, does not mean that our soul-path is going to be accepted with open arms from the rest of our 'earthly family'.

Key issues of this chakra are *survival and safety*. Contraction of this chakra can often be roused by just 'thinking about' what would happen if we were to 'go against the tide', thereby risking abandonment by our family or tribe. *How would we survive? Could we survive?* Further, do we feel a threat to our *safety* in any way? The issues of survival and safety are so basic for us that they create visceral reactions in the body when we perceive threats of any kind. In these instances, threats to our survival and safety can cause this chakra to contract to such an extent that we become incapable of moving forward physically, much less emotionally.

The legendary psychologist, Abraham Maslow (1908–1970) placed the human need for safety and security immediately above our basic physiological need for air, water, food and sleep (among others) in his famous 'Hierarchy of Needs'. Thus, our need for safety and security within family and tribe is paramount for us to function and survive in a chaotic world.*

A chronic state of contraction in the first chakra, triggered by emotions and feelings of fear for our survival, take

*http://web.utk.edu/~gwynne/maslow.htm.

a heavy toll on our immune system by shifting the chemistry in our body. The result is that our immune system eventually begins to deteriorate. Such shifts in our chemistry can
first appear as something mildly bothersome such as lower
back pain (no support there) escalating to psychological
depression (from mild to extreme) and/or life threatening
illnesses such as cancer and heart disease.

Once we discover the area of contraction, we can then
examine the remedies required to help our expansion. In
this case, *Walnut* is:

> *The Remedy for those who have decided to take a great step forward in life, to
> break old conventions, to leave old limits and restrictions and start on a new
> way ... a great spell-breaker, both of things of the past commonly called
> heredity, and circumstances of the present.**

While Bach considered Walnut the 'right remedy' for protecting us from unwanted outside influences, this was not
his only consideration in the application of Walnut. As we
can see from the above quotation, he also felt one could call
upon Walnut to assist us in breaking old patterns and what
can be considered 'toxic' ties.

The American author John Bradshaw, noted for his work
in interpersonal relationships, has used the phrase 'the ties
that bind' in reference to toxic relationships and circumstances in our lives that prevent us from manifesting our
highest potential. In terms of our spiritual path, such toxicity prevents us from moving forward toward discovering
our soul's fire.

When the root (first) chakra is in a contracted state, fam-
ily/tribal relationships by their very nature keep us tethered

*Chancellor, p. 201.

in an unhealthy way. In reality, they keep us so intimately and sometimes so cunningly bound, that we do not recognize they are the very source of our emotional impotence. This toxic binding can manifest in the co-dependent behaviour discussed in connection to *Centaury*, in Chapter Six. Moreover, because key issues of the root chakra are safety and survival, severing toxic ties for many seems out of the question. Furthermore, a contracted state of this chakra is a welcome breeding-ground for what the author Julia Cameron, who wrote *The Artist's Way*, calls 'crazy-makers'.

According to Cameron, crazy-makers 'are those personalities that create storm centres'. Among their behavioural characteristics, she includes their ability to break deals and destroy schedules, discount your reality, spending your time and money in the process. Furthermore, crazy-makers expect special treatment and they are expert blamers who hate order.† These individuals are so clever and believable that their appearance into our lives ultimately sets up an internal dialogue that blocks our ability to move forward.

As we will see a bit further on, crazy-makers not only lodge in our root chakra but they are part of our karmic contract. Although it may seem that their sole job is to deter us from discovering our soul's fire, the reality is that they are an important part of our growth dynamic. A key to our continued growth rests in the ways in which we respond to them and the situations they create for us. From a karmic

*'Crazy-makers' is a perfect description for the negative indication of Bach's White Chestnut remedy. While this particular remedy will not be discussed in these chapters, readers can refer to complete descriptions in any of the sources on the Bach remedies listed in 'Further Reading'. †Julia Cameron, *The Artist's Way*, 1992, p. 46–9.

perspective, crazy-makers are actually in our lives to test our mettle. Their unspoken question to us is, do we want to move forward on our soul-path, or take a pass, stay where we are, only to repeat the same script (albeit different cast), the next time around?

If we are able to come to the awareness that these elements in our lives are responsible for the contraction of our root chakra and the drain on our personal power, Walnut will help us confidently sever those binding ties that keep the lid on our stuckness. Walnut however, is not the only remedy that we need to consider in our root chakra first aid kit, which brings us to *Cherry Plum.*

Cherry Plum was the first remedy of the final nineteen that Bach discovered. He described Cherry Plum as the remedy for the mind being over-worked, unable to take 'strain'. Furthermore, he noted that one is in the 'negative' Cherry Plum state:

> *When impulses come upon us to do things we should not in the ordinary way think about or for one moment consider. The remedy for this comes from the Cherry Plum. . . . This drives away all the wrong ideas and* gives the sufferer mental strength and confidence.*

As a Registered Bach Foundation Practitioner, I am aware that each of the remedies has an extreme indication of its contracted state. For Cherry Plum, this state is contemplation of suicide. I have not only seen this emotional state in my clients, I have also seen the action of this remedy lift the fog of perception that the contracted Cherry Plum state manifests.

Essential keys in Cherry Plum issues are those of control

*Barnard, *Collected Writings*, p. 8 (author emphasis).

and internal struggle. Very often in my presentations on the remedies, I use Cherry Plum as an example of Bach's philosophy concerning conflict between the soul-agenda and the personality. In the contracted Cherry Plum state, the individual's internal struggle typically centres on a clash between external moral pressures (particularly in the family/tribe agendas) and internal emotions.

In these circumstances, the individual experiences the pressures of an environment that emphasizes order and mental rationale over the emotions of the soul's fire and happiness. In the more extreme circumstances forces within that environment can be abusive both emotionally and physically. We only have to look to some of the rigid cultural and religious frameworks that exist today as examples. Thus, the only avenue of escape open to these individuals is emotional shutdown. External characteristics that indicate such a state has occurred include irrational hysteria, temper tantrums, and even psychotic behaviour. Signs of depression are not unusual, and sometimes are seen in depressive behaviour: lack of sleep, hopelessness, or episodic outbursts of rage.

Unable to distinguish between the soul's intent and the moral expectations placed upon the soul and the personality by others, the individual can feel as if they are 'coming apart at the seams'. The contracted mood state of Cherry Plum is one that is very much about light and dark, according to Barnard.* Recalling Bach's words that the Cherry Plum remedy 'gives the sufferer mental strength and confidence', we can add it to our tool-kit for first-chakra contraction

*2003, p. 186.

should we 'feel' that this is the source of our stagnation.

As with all of the chakras, the ideal approach to taking inventory of 'how we are' is contemplative introspection, such as meditation. If we are not familiar with this method and find it difficult to practice in the beginning, we can always look to the body; listen to what the body is telling us and where. If we are honest with ourselves, the clues will rear up before us like red warning lights. Once we are able to recognize these clues, we can consider solutions and the remedies needed so that we can act upon our solutions with *Hope.*

CHAPTER TEN

PERSONAL BEST—CHOICE AND RESILIENCE: THE SECOND CHAKRA

Pine, Crab Apple—Peace

*A true shaman keeps no secrets about knowledge that can help and
heal. The difficulty is not in keeping knowledge secret, but in getting
people to understand and use it.... Widely spread knowledge actually
has more potency than secrets locked up and unused.... And the
sacredness of knowledge lies not in its reservation for a few, but in its
availability to many.... And finally, shamans recognize no hierarchy
or authority in matters of the mind; if ever a group of people could be
said to follow a system of spiritual democracy, it would be the shamans
of the world.*

SERGE KAHILI KING, PH.D., in *Urban Shaman*

WHETHER he was aware of it or not (and it is doubtful that
this was a conscious consideration) Edward Bach certainly
belongs in the realm of Shamanic healer* as well as that of
mystic.

*Shamanism is a healing tradition found in every major culture in the
world. It dates back at least 50,000 years, according to Dr Larry Dossey in his
article, 'When Stones Speak: Toward a Reenchantment of the World.' *Alternative
Therapies in Medicine and Health*, 2.4 (1996): 8–13, 97–103.

The Shaman in a community is the holistic healer, storyteller, priest, mystic, and psychotherapist, to name a few of his/her roles. Concerning matters of illness and death, Shamanism focuses on, and works in, the spiritual realms. For the Shaman, there are three main causes of illness. Two of these are loss of power and loss of soul. Loss of power essentially means that the power animal or spirit guardian, who has been protecting the individual from the spiritual plane, is no longer around him or her. This loss of power can manifest as 'chronic depression, chronic suicidal tendencies and chronic illness where a person can't seem to maintain his or her own immune system.'*

Loss of soul, or 'soul-loss', to a Shamanic healer means that a piece of the individual's life-force or vitality has escaped into space of 'non-ordinary reality'. Typically, this fragmentation is the result of some type of trauma or threat to the individual. When fragmentation occurs, the bit of life-force in question waits in safety for the Shaman to facilitate a reconnection to the body through a healing ritual known as 'soul-retrieval'. Further, according to the psychologist and author, Jeanne Achterberg: 'Soul loss is regarded as the gravest diagnosis in [Shamanism], being seen as a cause of illness and death. Yet it is not referred to at all in modern Western medical books.† Psychologists call the Shamanistic concept of 'fragmentation' by the term 'dissociation'.

Given that Bach had an interest in the beliefs and tradi-

---

*See Sandra Ingerman, MA, 'Medicine for the Earth, Medicine for People', *Alternative Therapies in Health and Medicine* 9.6 (2003): pp. 77–78. †Cameron, *The Vein of Gold*, New York, 1996, p. 78.

tions of other cultures, it is possible that he came across the subject of Shamanic healing. But whether he studied the fundamentals of Shamanism extensively is doubtful.* However, what *is* interesting is that in writing about the healing powers of the remedies, Bach continually speaks of their ability to give us courage so that we may realize our divinity; in other words, they empower us. Furthermore, on the subject of illness, Bach identified dissociation or disconnection between the soul and the personality (or what a Shaman might consider 'soul-loss') as the fundamental cause of illness.† Thus, however differently it is expressed, Bach's philosophy on illness and healing tracks interesting parallels with the philosophies of the healing traditions in Shamanism.

Although it is doubtful that the majority of us adhere to or practice in Shamanic traditions, understanding the concept of loss of power (disempowerment) and loss of soul (dissociation) is important. This is because as we continue in our process of emotional excavation, we find that contraction of the second chakra is about loss of our creative power. Moreover, depending on the extent of this loss, soul-fragmentation may be part of the picture as well. The second chakra is *the* gateway for our life-force and all forms of creativity. Given that life-force and the power of our creativity are inexorably linked, we can further consider that

---

*One of the world's foremost authorities on Shamanism, Mercia Eliade, was a contemporary of Bach's. However, all the indications are that Eliade's extensive works on the subject were not published until after Bach's death. It is possible however, that Bach may have come across some of Eliade's early writings that were in anticipation of his future works on the subject of Shamanism and religious philosophy in general. †Barnard, *Collected Writings*, p. 129.

any impediment to this union has a powerful impact on any progress we make on our spiritual path.

Additionally, the health of the second chakra profoundly affects the activity or inactivity of the other chakras. When expanded, this chakra is a vibrant core of the emotional and spiritual energy that fires our power of choice. This expansion also provides us with resilience from decisions that we have made that play out in every relationship of our lives. When the second chakra is in a state of expansion, we are in full ownership of our creative selves. Conversely, when this chakra contracts, power of choice is not an option and we are critically dis-empowered and emotionally disabled. Thus, in our disempowerment, our fear of the loss of control translates into intense attempts *to control* our internal and immediate external environment. With a second chakra shut down, vital life-force from the Divine cannot enter and this leads to stagnation and erratic functioning of the other six centres. Physical difficulties relating to sexual health, or problems with our reproductive organs such as prostate or ovarian cancer and menopausal difficulties, including fibroid cysts, all point to stagnant-energy issues in this chakra. Chronic lower back issues, colon, and hip areas also are an indication of second-chakra contraction.

In addition, the second chakra is the unconscious dumping-ground for all of our unresolved fears that have to do with relationships. Myss states that within the diverse symptomology of a malfunctioning second chakra, fear of betrayal and loss are primary issues. These can materialize in a myriad of scenarios that involve money, sex, loss of power, control, rape (emotionally and physically) or abandonment, to name a few.* As spirit in body, the fabric of our emotions and feelings is a complex weave. Life in the body is difficult; relationships are difficult and it is here, particularly in our second chakra, that our soul-lessons concerning the power of choice and relationships play out energetically and spiritually.

Karmically speaking, each of us carries some history of betrayal. Nevertheless, when betrayal is a major theme for us, particularly in the area of personal relationships, our individual behaviour can lead to dysfunctional control issues. Internally, we may experience mild to extreme anxiety if we feel we are not in control of the environment around us. Externally we can become victims of social phobia or the more extreme version, agoraphobia. One who experiences the dynamics of these disorders is unable to socialize well, and may be unable to do so altogether. For example, agoraphobics can become so emotionally paralyzed, that they cannot even leave their homes. Externally, and at the other end of the spectrum, their internal fear of losing control translates into extreme control behaviour that is dictatorial in its interaction with everything and everyone around them. Sadly, this behaviour leads to disconnection from others and possibly, disassociation; surely a lonely existence. At the root of the betrayal theme lie emotional issues of guilt, shame, and an internal message of self-deprecation that tells us erroneously that we are undeserving of making choices. Clearly, if one is functioning in a state of shame or guilt, there is little hope of capturing or manifesting the soul's desired path.

*Myss, *Anatomy*, p. 130.

When they feel hypercritical, all environments (including parenting, partnerships, cultural, and religious models that are part of our everyday 'reality) ignite second-chakra issues. As we noted in Chapter Three, the 'holy anorexia' that manifested in medieval nuns is a perfect example of internal control issues within an extremely controlling religious environment. Within our framework of the remedies, this behaviour is a reactive 'lashing out' of an extreme contracted Pine state. Nevertheless, the 'crazy-makers' who are part of these landscapes, are a 'soul set-up', giving us the opportunity to overcome these obstacles so that we can retrieve the power we are meant to have. If we continually experience outcomes in our relationships wherein others ignore our needs and our dreams are shattered, we feel *betrayed*.

Because of these feelings, we have a built-in internal warning mechanism that triggers 'red flags'. Through these experiences, our soul is sending us a very strong message: Take responsibility! It is urging us to take a personal inventory and ascertain our contributions to the relationships that continually create disappointing scenarios. Nevertheless, with a contracted second chakra, taking an objective inventory is a tough assignment, because this process potentially brings to light additional self-deprecation and emotional distress that we must examine in order to determine how we arrived at this 'place'.

A more obvious approach at this point may be to check in with our physical wellbeing. If we are emotionally or mentally unaware that there is contracted energy in this chakra, our body certainly has many ways to raise red flags. In the Bach repertoire, *Pine* and *Crab Apple* are two remedies that have a compelling ability to shift individual perception from disempowerment to empowerment, even when our choices do not produce the expected outcome.

A constricted emotional Pine state is one that is reflected in shame-based guilt. In this state, one operates from a core of unworthiness, simply by being in the body. From day one in this incarnation, the contracted Pine mood-state or personality-type feels and believes that they are unworthy. They tend to ruminate over what they have done, did not do, should have done or said. Additionally, individuals stuck in the second chakra who are manifesting the constricted Pine state will often take on the responsibility for another's dysfunction; 'it's my fault' is their chronic internal and external dialogue.

Unfortunately, repetitive episodes of betrayal that these individuals experience reinforce this belief. Furthermore, because they are laden with shame and guilt, they believe that they are always the problem and always the reason behind these episodes. It is doubtful that this assessment is accurate, but in their minds, it is and therefore, they can never do enough or say enough. In a phrase, they will 'never be enough' and this belief leads to additional dysfunctional forms of behaviour.

If we can momentarily set Pine aside, the remedy Crab Apple with its similarities to, and the very subtle differences from, the contracted Pine state is worthy of valuable consideration. For Bach, the Crab-Apple remedy was the remedy of 'purification'.* Its constricted state in many ways is similar to the constricted Pine state when lodged in the second

*Barnard, 2002, p. 229.

chakra, in that both have to do with shame and guilt. However, the shame of Crab Apple manifests in the belief of not being internally clean enough. Thus, in this constricted state, there is an intense belief of internal self-disgust.

Evidence of the constricted Crab Apple state in the second chakra usually surfaces through specific issues of cleanliness and sexual dysfunction that can manifest in obsessive behaviour. It is not unusual for an individual stuck in the constricted Crab Apple state to become so fixated on some insignificant physical impurity (usually having to do with the skin), that they totally miss a more serious health issue. When the second chakra is constricted and the Crab Apple remedy is indicated, there is an underlying belief held by the individual that there is some poison present that must be eradicated from the body. The problem is that as long as the constriction remains, the expulsion is never complete. Furthermore, the belief surrounding impurity totally blocks the infusion of spiritual light and creativity into this chakra. Sexually this constriction can manifest in impotence, frigidity or a general belief that sexual enjoyment is 'dirty behaviour' or 'sinful'.

Ironically, the constricted states of both Pine and Crab Apple typically manifest in the drive for perfection and over achievement. Examples of extremes in these dynamics are prominent in the behaviours found in people who suffer from the eating disorders known as Anorexia Nervosa and Bulimia.*

---

*Mack, Gaye. 'Exploring Implications of Treating Eating Disorders with Vibrational Medicine as an Integrative Therapy'. 1999, DePaul University, Chicago, Illinois.

As I mentioned in earlier chapters, while Bach considered that the Twelve Healers represented soul-types and their lessons, he later recognized that the Twelve Healers also represented personality-types and temporary mood-states as well. As an example of this interconnection between all of the thirty-eight remedies, we can also look to the zealous contraction of Vervain and its relationship to the obsessive, controlling behaviour of contracted Pine and Crab Apple. As the Pine and Crab-Apple contracted states escalate in their drive to over-achieve and in their anxiety to control, they further take on the contracted state of Vervain that can be intensely zealous and fanatical. The difference here is that the *root* of Vervain is enthusiasm, while the *roots* of Pine and Crab Apple are guilt and shame. In the contracted Pine and Crab-Apple states, it is a question of the *type* of guilt/shame. For those in the contracted Pine state, it is about *what they have done;* for those in the contracted Crab Apple state, it is about *who they are.* Frequently, an individual will manifest both of these contracted states simultaneously.

It is worth noting that perhaps Bach had a particular relationship to Pine. We know from Nora Weeks that Bach experienced the contracted emotional states of each of the final nineteen remedies just prior to their discovery. Furthermore, we also know from Weeks that he worked in his father's foundry for three years with some difficulty, before approaching his father on the subject attending medical school. Weeks reports that behind this delay in expressing his desire to study medicine, was the feeling that he could not ask his parents for the necessary funds required.* Why

*Weeks, *Discoveries*, p. 12–13.

was this? Barnard speculates that as the oldest son, perhaps
Bach thought he should go into the family business. If this
were the case, and he was finding it difficult to separate from
this expectation, aspects of Walnut (as discussed in Chapter
Nine) are evident. Here, however, it seems that there is more
between the lines in Bach's personal history. In *Heal Thyself,*
Bach takes issue with the nature of parenting:

> *The whole attitude of parents should be to give the little newcomer all the*
> *spiritual, mental and physical guidance to the utmost of their ability, ever*
> *remembering that the wee one is an individual soul come down to gain his own*
> *experience and knowledge in this own way according to the dictates of his*
> *Higher Self, and every possible freedom should be given for unhampered de-*
> *velopment.* *

He later seems to reiterate his beliefs on the subject of
parenting in *Free Thyself* using a somewhat stronger voice:

> *So many suppress their real desires and become square pegs in round holes:*
> *through the wishes of a parent, a son may be come a solicitor, a soldier, a*
> *business man, when his true desire is to become carpenter. . . . This sense of*
> *duty is then a false sense of duty, and a dis-service to the world; it results in*
> *unhappiness and, probably, the greater part of a lifetime wasted before the*
> *mistake can be rectified.* †

Clearly, Bach was addressing, in so many words, the second-chakra issue of empowerment through choice; and
equally importantly, our ability to embrace resilience from
our choices regardless of the ramifications. Bach himself
possessed an intensive drive for completing tasks that in
some respects was obsessive. Furthermore, this behaviour
and his recurring theme of life and soul-path choices, indicates that Pine and second chakra issues were significant for

---

*Barnard, *Collected Writings*, p. 138. †Barnard, *Collected Writings*, p. 97.

him on a deeply personal level. For him, his writings were a vehicle through which he could safely express the dissatisfactions and frustrations that were part of his own personal history. Here again is a subtle reminder that although he was brilliantly gifted and a mystic, Bach, like the rest of us, was challenged by his own personal dragons.

On our own journey, it is important that we examine how we make our choices and the reasons behind making the decisions that we do. We need to keep in mind that this is a second-chakra issue and that the second chakra is the seat of our creative energy. While constriction of this chakra impedes the flow of creativity, we can call upon the remedies of Pine and Crab Apple to assist us. As the remedies aid our ability to shift our emotional energy and perspective, we have the opportunity to discover our power of choice and resilient strength. Moreover, with these, we are able to embrace a sense of internal *peace* with our decisions in the knowledge that we are free to make different choices.

CHAPTER ELEVEN

SOLAR POWER: THE THIRD CHAKRA

Larch, Willow & Holly—Joy

'*No one can make you feel inferior without your consent*'
ELEANOR ROOSEVELT

WITH THE third chakra, we come to the last centre of the lower triangle in our chakra symbology of the inverted triangles. In the 'last but not least' category, its placement is far from insignificant, as we make our way upwards into the upper triangle. Located in what is known as the solar plexus of our body, this chakra is the seat of our internal self-command of our exterior environment. This is where our conscious 'fire' resides. It is this fire that we need in order for us to progress forward when faced with karmic challenges along our soul-path. As the centre of the normal feelings and emotions, this is where we consciously experience everyday life—through our joys, desires, anger, ambitions, anxieties, and/or fears of failure and success. Finally, this centre represents the alchemical melting-pot or union of the expanded authority achievable in our first and second centres.

As I described in Chapters Nine and Ten, the first and second chakras represent the fostering of healthy ties within the greater collective and the realization that exercising the power of choice is necessary in order to follow our intended soul-path. It is important for us to remember, also, that separation from the 'tribe' or tribal ways is sometimes necessary for us to move forward. Furthermore, in any such separation we are propelled into activating the power of choice that we are entitled to as individual souls.

In Chapter Six, it was put forward that Dr Bach believed each of us has incarnated in this life with a soul-lesson to transform. By working to shift the hindrance of our particular lesson into its quality or virtue, we have the opportunity to offer the benefits of its virtue to other human beings. The intensity and harmony of our third-chakra fire depends on how well we have learned to balance the emotional patterns of the tribal male energy of the first chakra and the creative feminine energy of our second chakra. Determining our progress in the expansion of the first two chakras is vital because this progress has a direct impact on our sense of self and the contributions we can make to our external environment and the world.

As with of each of the chakra centres, formidable challenges face us in the third chakra. Third-chakra issues include sensitivity to external critics, invalidation by others, lack of self-esteem, and the inability to trust our intuitive voice, which is the voice of our soul. Thus, our work is cut out for us as we discover that this chakra involves both internal and external development.

In Chapter Four, we met the concept of the 'hungry ghost', described by psychologist, Jack Kornfield. The hungry ghost that resides in each of us is our chronic wanting; if we only had more, we could do more, be more. On our mystic path, we discover that our wanting can fuel our solar fire either positively or negatively and that the third chakra is the battleground of these polarities. The emotional experiences we have with our external and internal environment reflect the degree of success or failure in this challenge. The question becomes, how do these reflections manifest?

We find that the core health of this centre emotionally, physically, and spiritually, is reflected in the security we experience through our self-esteem, or alternatively in the lack of it. As Caroline Myss observes, 'No one is born with healthy self-esteem. We must earn this quality in the process of living as we face our challenges one at a time.*

Thus, we need to remember that on the spiritual level, we attract relationships and circumstances that give us opportunities to transform contracted states of our chakras into states of expansion. When our third centre is contracted our self-esteem is weak and, for some of us, totally nonexistent. In this contracted state, there is lack of self-confidence as well as a lack of an ability to succeed in the external world. We are unaware that we are compromised, because we easily defer to others—believing they are smarter, more experienced, have more talent, are more creative. In a simple phrase, *they are more and we are invisible.* The reality is that in our deferment, we have abdicated not only our personal power, but also our divinity.

However, deferment is not the only manifestation of a weakened self-esteem. Just as easily as we defer, we can also

*Anatomy, p. 169.

go on the attack, full of fiery acrimonious energy. This energy can fuel attitudes and actions of arrogance, intimidation, self-righteousness, and abusive anger; or we can simply be obnoxiously opinionated. Regardless of which of the many exterior expressions our weakened self-esteem takes, they are always about dumping our toxic emotions on others. *They all mask a gut fear of 'not being'* and a fear that we are fated to be swallowed up by our environment. In addition, third-chakra contraction prevents access to our intuition and blocks 'soul-messages' from coming through. It skews our perceptions. Through the lens of our hypersensitivity, we misinterpret innocuous remarks and behaviour by others. Constructive observations, suggestions, even innocent humour, and behaviour all translate as criticism intended to spotlight our self-assigned lack of intelligence and abilities. Thus, feeling invalidated by the external world, we protect our secret of low or nonexistent self-esteem through misguided reactions.

Contracted, the fire of the third chakra fans the flames of rage and anger shrouded in verbal lashings or recriminations spewed out toward others. In more extreme reactions, physical vindictiveness may emerge. In any case, all of these responses are smokescreens for shame of inadequacy. Further, such behaviour carries a double-edged sword. At the very least, it most certainly hurts those who become targets. Furthermore, it also carries the potential of relationships being severed altogether. Thus, leaving a trail of relationship ashes, we can move from one encounter to the next, never clearly understanding 'what happened'. The irony is that those with whom we respond to most negatively, whether it be with arrogance, intimidation, self-righteousness or abuse, are the very individuals our soul has chosen to help us to strengthen our self-esteem and value.

Energetically, the third chakra centre is where we assimilate either healthy or unhealthy energy from our environment. It is also where we may 'leak' the energy needed to discover our soul's fire and manifest it. We are spirit in body, but from the physical perspective the impact of third-chakra contraction is enormous. As the solar plexus is the gravitational centre of our body, imbalance in this centre is a tenuous two-way street. Physical manifestations include difficulties with the upper intestine, abdominal area, liver, gallbladder, adrenals, spleen and mid spine.*

From an Ayurvedic perspective,†

the intestinal tract is at the centre of the organizational plan that governs human functions. It is the crux of the matter. This notion is echoed in other traditions, too.... There seems to be a sort of consensus that it is here where health is rooted and where disease originates.§

To Ayurvedic and other holistic practitioners, the state of our emotions is a vital variable in the overall picture of our harmony. If our emotions are not at peace, particularly in the third chakra, we can easily move into a state of dysbiosis, i.e., disorder in the intestinal tract. As a bacteriologist, Edward Bach repeatedly wrote about the necessity of intestinal cleanliness.¤ Perhaps it was from examining the philosophies of the East that he came to subscribe to this belief. However, it is not only our intestinal health that is at risk when our third centre is contracted. It is often said that the

---

*Anatomy, p. 96. †Ayurveda is the ancient system of holistic medicine originating in India. §Ballantine, p. 249. ¤Barnard, 2002, p. 229.

liver is the seat of unresolved anger that smoulders and that we 'vent' anger through our spleen. Furthermore, negative emotions drain energy from our adrenals. Overall, any of these unhealthy conditions are catalysts for a depleted immune system. It is a downwards spiral and whether we regain or do not regain vigorous health may depend on its severity. Unfortunately, from the spiritual plane, when we ignore soul-signals and messages, the Divine will bring us to our knees through the only vehicle that we seem to understand at this point, and that is our body.

It is important to make mention here of the fact that in many new-age circles there is a philosophy that illness and disease are a form of punishment foisted upon us by 'spirit'. This punitive belief is in direct contrast to Bach's beliefs and writings:

> It matters not our stage of advancement, whether aborigine or disciple, is of no consequence as regards health; but what is important is that we, whatever our station, live in harmony with the dictates of our soul. . . . During our sojourn in search of perfection, there are various stages . . . and we have to master stage by stage as we progress. Some stages may be comparatively easy, some exceedingly difficult, and then it is that disease occurs, because it is at those times that we fail to follow our Spiritual Self, that the conflict arises which produces illness.

Thus, according to Bach, illness is not a matter of punishment, but a matter of notification that we are not 'listening'.

Recalling that the different permutations of the thirty-eight remedies number in the hundreds of millions, we find that various aspects of each remedy are effective in addressing forms of chakra contraction. As an example, we can

*Barnard, *Collected Writings*, p. 158.

consider Pine and Crab Apple in connection with the 'shame' aspect found in this centre. Additionally, practitioners traditionally use Walnut to help protect and seal the solar plexus from unwanted energy assimilation and drain. There are also three additional remedies that are particularly useful for the maladies we can experience from contraction in this centre.

Larch is *the* remedy Bach identified for issues of self-esteem. As the lack of self-esteem is the core emotion driving contraction in our third centre, Larch is extremely important. Recalling Myss' statement that self-esteem is not something we are born with, but rather something that we must earn, the contracted third chakra that is mirrored by the negative Larch state is one that is a result of life and/or relationship difficulties. Similar to Pine and Crab Apple, negative Larch is possibly the result of the individual having to endure years of harsh criticism, belittlement, or lack of encouragement and support. Thus, there is little desire to extend to the outside world, as the internal belief is that failure is a probable outcome, no matter what is attempted. In the extreme of lacking self-confidence, such an individual will not even try because they *know* they will fail. Larch as a remedy in one's formula* works to bolster self-confidence by shifting the perception into one that aids us in the understanding that each of us is blessed with divine gifts that are unique and meant to be contributed to benefit those around us. However, while self-confidence is the core issue in third-chakra contraction, we also need remedies that will

*Refer to 'Practical Matters' at the end of this book for information on creating a 'personal remedy formula'.

assist in shifting the negative behaviour through which we express this shame.

As I noted earlier, smouldering, unresolved anger can be deadly to us on a physical level, especially in matters involving the liver. This makes sense since the liver is the organ responsible for detoxifying our body. The holistic author, Louise Hay, identifies cancer in general as the manifestation of long-held resentment eating away at us internally.* From a chakra perspective, we are reminded by both of the authors I have mentioned—Myss and Hay—that holistic philosophy in general identifies unresolved emotional issues 'stuck' in a particular chakra through the physical location of illness points. According to Dr Bach, the remedy needed for resentment, bitterness and/or self-pity is *Willow*. In the contracted emotional state, the Willow mood† exhibits any or all of these particular emotions. Typically, those who are in a contracted Willow state point the finger of blame at everyone and everything else as being the source of their problems. The subtle message behind this state is that the individual never 'owns' their participation or non-participation in their situation. This contraction is most likely a carry-over from contraction issues of shame and guilt in the second chakra, thus compounding the situation. Unable to access the energy needed to transform their compromised self-esteem, they simply cannot get to the point where they can understand that in taking some degree of responsibility for their actions they are on their way to enhancing their self-esteem.

*Hay, p. 12. †Interestingly, Bach did not identify Willow as also being a personality type.

Several years ago, a psychotherapist and I shared a client who was in a contracted Willow state. Working as a part-time nurse, with two children under the age of five and a husband who travelled constantly, she was someone who clearly had a lot on her plate. Over the course of many months, the therapist and I worked with various remedy-combinations to help this woman with the obsessive-compulsive behaviours she was using as a form of self-medication. *

On the surface, the client never verbally expressed resentment of her situation or blame; in fact, it was quite the opposite. Raised in the strict Catholic tradition, she bore her situation with an air that sometimes resembled martyrdom. However it wasn't until she became pregnant with her third child that she began to lament the situation in which she had obviously participated and I realized I was seeing the contracted Willow state. I immediately stopped her current formula and suggested Willow by itself. Being a very compliant individual, the client began taking the Willow immediately and within forty-eight hours was on the phone to her therapist crying in the realization that 'she had been setting [herself] up for self-sabotage all of these years'.

It is interesting to note that the negative Willow state has an aspect of inflexibility or resistance about it, through the refusal to take responsibility for oneself. Conversely, the remedy brings flexibility to the individual through the will-

---

*Bach believed the process of harmonizing our emotions required not just one remedy, but often a combination of remedies. As such, the combination an individual might begin with changes as the emotions shift in their harmonization. This process is often referred to in practice as a 'peeling of the onion'.

ingness to participate in his/her process and the awareness of how this process fits into the overall picture of his/her intended soul-path. It is also important to note that it is rare for the remedies to work so quickly when there are deep-seated issues involved. In this case, however, it is likely that subconsciously her misery was so intense that she was at a point where she was ready to participate in her 'excavation' at a deeper level. Thus, the Willow acted as a catalyst in bring-ing her to the awareness that *her own* actions were, in great part, behind her misery. With the help of her therapist and additional formula-combinations, she was ready to address the contracted issues of shame and disempowerment lodged in her second chakra as well.

As I noted earlier, the destructive emotions of anger and rage are not always repressed. We can see, unfortunately, an explosion of these unrepressed emotions being expressed around the globe. This all-too-prevalent 'in your face' rage camouflages contracted third-chakra compromised self-es-teem. It is critical to remember that this type of anger is al-ways abusive and is an indication that the remedy *Holly* is necessary. As a personality or mood-state, the Holly type was placed by Bach in his category *Over-Sensitive to Influences and Ideas*. The behaviour of the contracted Holly state sub-ject is very serious because it is mirrored in all forms of abuse. Whether it comes out emotionally or physically, the Holly state is violent; it is simply a matter of degree. In the ex-treme contraction, this state is vindictive, hell-bent on re-venge. The irony is that the Holly 'personality' is actually very sensitive and has suffered some form of abuse in this life, past lives or both. This reinforces what psychologists know from experience: 'the abuser has been the abused'. Thus, lacking the experience of love, with little or no self-esteem, these individuals 'keep score' of each perceived cruelty they have experienced. Internally there is an intense, unhealthy 'burning' that can drive them to lose control and into a protective behavioural mode of 'payback'. Bach established that those individuals exhibiting the negative Holly state or personality-type suffer a great deal internally 'often when there is no real cause for their unhappiness'.*

In this observation of Bach's we are again informed that negative emotions have an effect upon our perceptions. To re-emphasize this: when we experience the energy of negative emotions, this experience fuels contraction in our chakras. At the same time, our perceptions of our environment become skewed and highly inaccurate. The action of the remedies assists in shifting our perceptions from unreality to the reality around us. Because of their own history of abuse, whether it be emotional, physical or both, an individual in the contracted Holly state perceives that everyone is 'out to get them'. This state can only escalate unless they call upon tools that will help them to neutralize these perceptions. If this state is chronic, there is an indication that the individual is carrying baggage of a very difficult history and, typically, such individuals are in need of some type of psychotherapy. With therapeutic assistance and the assistance of the remedy Holly (and others), perceptions become more balanced, moving into reality. Through this process, those who have had to struggle are now able to step back and view their experience through a clearer and more real-

*Barnard, Collected Writings, p. 42.

istic lens. Simultaneously, the third chakra begins to expand, self-esteem builds, and awareness of soul-path becomes *their* reality and their *joy* in being engaged in the world.

We now move into the upper triangle of our chakra symbology, beginning with the Fourth Chakra, that of the Heart. It is further important to re-emphasize that working with the contracted states of the first three chakra centres is vital if we intend to embrace fully our intent to discover our soul's fire. As Caroline Myss states:

not only do we want to 'know about' . . . reincarnation, meditation, and spiritual ecstasy, we want to 'live' them. We want power of these spiritual teachings to activate our biological tissue; we want to feel the presence of God in our bodies as well as in our minds. We want physical contact with the Divine, matching the level of contact previously enjoyed by saints and mystics of the great tradition.*

In order to reach this goal, in order to discover our soul's fire, we first need to 'chop wood, carry water'. In other words, we need to *work* at the mundane everyday chores that keep us going and do not appear glamorous. This means showing up, paying attention to what is going on within us at ground level, and excavating toxic emotions. These are necessary keys to the experience of *joy*. Moreover, they are necessary before we can ascend upwards into the ethers.

*Myss, *Why People don't Heal,* pp. 86–7.

CHAPTER TWELVE

AT THE CROSSROADS—STATE OF THE HEART: THE FOURTH CHAKRA

Beech, Honeysuckle, Star of Bethlehem—Unconditional Love

In Egyptian mythology, there is the general myth that upon death, an individual's heart was weighed by Anubis against the goddess Maat's feather. If the heart was heavy as a result of foul thoughts and actions, it would outweigh the feather, and the soul would be fed to the shadow world. But if the scales were balanced, indicating that the heart of the deceased was pure in intent and that the individual had been just and honourable in life, he would be welcomed by the god Osiris and passage into the sacred land offered.

BACK IN Chapter One is where we began our exploration with our image of standing on the platform waiting for the spiritual train. This platform is the place from where we peered at the constricted emotional patterns of the root, sacral, and solar plexus chakras. It is here that we were presented with a view of the karmic hindrances and emotional dragons that have the power to keep us emotionally 'stuck'. While these emotional hindrances and dragons may be intimidating, we explored the channels of expansion and growth that are possible with the help of several of the remedies. It is on this same platform that we now find ourselves faced with a decision. Even if we have been able to face the dragons of the lower centres, the question before us is, do we have the courage to do the work required for expansion in the lower three chakras? The answer to this question is the key to the quality of our process. Doing the emotional excavation of our lower three centres *is an absolute prerequisite to boarding the spiritual train that will take us further along the path to discovering our soul's fire and purpose.* The emotional patterns of our lower three centres are of the mundane world. But, if we are able to shift the contracted patterns of these centres, we have a precious opportunity to journey from the mundane to the wisdom of our spiritual heart and the wisdom of, in Bach's words, 'the Lord Buddha and other great Masters, who have come down from time to time upon earth to point out to men [and women] the way to attain perfection.' First, however, we must decide which emotional pattern will be the model for our progress on our mystic path. Will it be the consciousness of constriction held in our lower three chakras, or will it be the consciousness of expansion in these centres?

This dilemma returns us to our spot on the spiritual platform where we found ourselves in Chapter One: are we willing to climb on board with our karmic baggage in order to discover our soul's fire? While we may have become aware of the work necessary for soul-growth, we tend to hear a small voice that says to us, 'This platform is the safe place; here, I don't have to commit to doing any new emotional work'. Here, one more time, we come face to face with our internal crazy-maker and the recurring theme of *choice.*

As I have made clear in previous chapters, our soul has

mapped out an agenda for us when we incarnate into this
life. Moreover, contained within this agenda is the challenge
for us to love unconditionally. As we study the beginning of
the upper triangle of our chakra symbology, much to our
surprise, we find that the emotions are the boarding pass
for the spiritual train and the heart is the gatekeeper. Thus,
we have come to the heart of what matters; it is this fourth
chakra centre that represents our balance between body (below) and spirit (above). In other words, 'Heart' matters in
all things physical, emotional, and spiritual. Physically, our
heart is responsible for keeping us alive in the body, for when
our heart fails, our body fails. Spiritually, it represents the
seat of our innate wisdom. It is our spiritual anchor and
record-keeper. However, access to this centre and our soul-
path is not easy and is often a struggle to obtain.

The heart chakra's vibrant emotional and spiritual energy of unconditional love holds the space for us as we experience the baptism of the four elements through the
emotional dragons discussed in Chapter Four. As our record-
keeper, it holds the remembrances of the joys, pleasures,
and moments of happiness, that we experience. But it also
holds the records of the sorrows, hurts and grievances that
can catapult us right back down into the contraction of those
dragons dwelling in the lower three centres. The choice is
ours as to where *we* are going to 'live'.

We must keep in mind that no matter how much sacred
shopping we have done and are still doing, in order to truly be
on our mystic path, we must make our way into the heart
chakra from the lower three chakras. In other words, we do
not just decide, 'oh, ok, if I think about loving uncondition-

ally, I am living it; I don't need to deal with all of that unpleasant emotional stuff. The temptation to intellectualize *our work* is without a doubt, the 'Venus Flytrap' on our mystical path.*

The caveat on our journey is that no matter how hard we try to utilize the intellectual route to become 'spiritual', it will not work. Energetically and emotionally, access to the heart wisdom is proportional to the expanded or contracted state of each of the lower chakras. As these centres are balanced, the heart expands, supporting the ongoing growth of the upper chakra centres. The heart centre is 'the centre where we learn to harmonize all the conflicting elements in our nature—all conflicts of mind or emotion'.† It is where we are learning the lesson of the Aquarian Age, the lesson of universal brotherhood; and it is a lesson that is *felt*, not *thought about*. The heart chakra as the gatekeeper is the centre that is affected by the state of the other centres. Conversely, it also affects the state of the other centres as well. If the heart centre is constricted, this has a direct constrictive effect upon the centres 'below' and the centres 'above'. Additionally, if the heart centre is expanded, it *supports* the expansion of the other centres as well. Thus like the image of mercury's fluidity referred to in Chapter Seven, there is an ongoing flow of energy upwards and downwards, expansive and contractive.

The expression, 'when your heart speaks, take good notes', is wise advice, for to do otherwise will result in emotional and physical dyspepsia. When contracted, the heart chakra is the

*In botany, 'the leaves of Venus Flytrap open wide and on them are short, stiff hairs called trigger or sensitive hairs. When anything touches these hairs enough to bend them, the two lobes of the leaves snap shut, trapping whatever is inside' (www.botany.org). †Hodgson, *Stars and Chakras,* p. 134.

unconscious dumping ground for the toxic emotions stuck
in the lower three centres: anger, rage, distrust, loneliness,
hatred, resentment and bitterness, to name a few.

There are volumes written on the dysfunctional ramifications of this particular chakra, but at the source of all of
these difficult emotions, lies grief. The experience of grief
tells us that something that has been lost. From the spiritual perspective, our primary grief is in our original separation from our Divinity. Thus, the humanness of the emotions with which we struggle is part of the necessary process
in reconnecting to our Divinity, or our higher self. Grief is
always an emotional challenge, but what is difficult for us
to grasp is that it is part of our expansion process. When we
are 'in grief', we are in an intensely painful process; we are *in
it* as a therapist friend of mine says. Moreover, it is a state
that *feels* so contracted that we cannot imagine that we will
ever come through it to the other side. However, the only
way out *is through*. In other words, in order to move forward
on our mystic path, we must be willing to acknowledge our
grief and then be willing to let it go honestly, rather than
hang onto it as an excuse for not manifesting our intended
path. Grief is a powerful messenger for us. It is the messenger that tells us, yes, there is loss. Nevertheless, if we honour the process and move through it, it is the spiritual messenger telling us that the universe waits with an abundance
of new possibilities and opportunities for us and then there
is *expansion!*

The manifestations of emotions connected to the grieving process are powerful and can easily lead to physical fall-
out. Thus, staying 'stuck' in our grief, commands a high

price, both emotionally and physically. Heart-chakra mal-functions are identified by Myss as any physical manifesta-tions affecting the lungs, breasts, diaphragm, and of course, the heart itself. Congestive heart failure, heart attacks, al-lergies, pneumonia, bronchitis, and breast cancer,* all point to contractions of this chakra as do the emotional expres-sions, 'heartless', 'heart-sick', and 'heartbroken'.

If we refer back to Chapters Ten and Eleven, wherein we looked at the emotional profiles and remedy characteristics of Pine, Crab Apple, Willow, Holly and Larch, we can see that the healing dynamics of these remedies can also be con-sidered for working with heart chakra issues. While this con-sideration once again demonstrates the adaptability of Dr Bach's thirty-eight remedies, we can explore two additional remedies at this point.

In lectures, when I speak about the remedy *Beech*, I de-scribe the emotional contraction of the Beech personality or mood state by using the phrase, 'beech bitches', which is the American vernacular that uses 'bitch' as a verb. True to form, this personality-type or mood-state does just this; it 'bitches'. In this state, the Beech personality sees an exter-nal environment that is inexcusably imperfect. For them their experience of the external environment is the unreal-ity of the reality. Their view through such a distorted lens generates behaviour that is judgmental, intolerant, and highly critical of everyone and everything around them—and they keep score of every infraction they perceive directed toward them, in a way similar to constricted Holly.

Their way of being becomes so narrow that they create

*Myss, *Anatomy*, p. 98.

their own constrictions in the way they function in life and
in their relationships with others. Seeking exactness and
perfection of others in ways that are unrealistic, they invite
isolation into their lives that is one more self-destructive
dynamic. 'If only the world and everyone in it would adhere to the way it should be', is the contracted Beech mantra.
Here again are clues to constricted third-chakra issues as
well. Simply, if we believe that we do not possess self-worth,
it is impossible for us to honour the worth in others; the shame
is too great, or we just do not see the worth in others.

Because they are unable to lessen their perception of flaws,
instead of recognizing what is glorious, this narrow way of
being can only affect the state of the heart with an eventual
outcome of illness. In cardiac health, it is interesting to consider the parallel between a narrow way of being and a nar-
rowing of the arteries, which in turn constricts the flow of
the blood: the carrier of our life's vitality on the physical level.

The positive energy or vibrations of the remedy Beech,
however, act as catalysts in assisting these individuals in the
transformation of their vision. Beech shifts the contracted
perception of judgment and intolerance to one that supports the expansion of the heart chakra and thus, expansion of the lower centres. Again, it is important to keep in
mind that on our mystic path, *everything* is interconnected;
what affects one chakra, affects them all. Finally, Bach's
philosophy on the contracted Beech state was this:

> *It is obvious that none of us is in a position to judge or criticize, for the wisest
> of us sees and knows only the minutest fragment of the Great Scheme of all
> things, and we cannot judge, knowing so little, how the Great Plan will work.*

As I stated earlier in this chapter, although the emotion of grief is a difficult one, it is a necessary part of the human process in soul-growth. Grief is *the* emotion that teaches us to *feel.* This does not mean that we are comfortable with this lesson. Most of us are not. Further, we do not always know that we are *in* grief or that we are grieving. The state of grieving that is most familiar to us is the intense sadness that overwhelms us at a time of loss, repeatedly telling others and ourselves that we are 'grieving'. However, being 'in grief' is a much longer process altogether. As an example, one who is 'in grief' may not be aware that they are in grief. The manifestation of such behaviours as anger, rage, and mild to extreme depression, eating disorders, and sexual dysfunction or sleep disorders, can indicate the state of grief in addition to the sadness that we connect with grief. Even if we are not able to identify these emotions as part of this process, we *know* that at some level we hurt.

While there are several remedies within the thirty-eight that are well suited to working with aspects of grief, two are of particular note: *Honeysuckle* and *Star of Bethlehem.*

Traditionally, practitioners consider Honeysuckle for the state of mind in which an individual cannot get out of the past. In other words, they may long for it (which is a form of grieving) or for someone who has passed over, recalling only pleasant memories that are far more comforting than they *actually* were, or their present reality. This mood state becomes particularly common as we age. Statements such as 'I remember when we....', 'Things were so much better back then', 'I don't know what has happened to the world, it was never like this' are all indications of contracted Honeysuckle.

*Chancellor, p. 46.

However, there is another hue to this mood, and it has to do with emotional wounding and the grief it creates. Some years ago, I had a psychotherapist tell me that, in her opinion, emotional wounds went far deeper than physical wounds. She went on to say that physical wounds could heal; often the emotional wounds stay with us for this lifetime and into the next.

Earlier I mentioned the term Caroline Myss uses for the attitude that keeps us stuck in our history, 'woundology'. She says, 'I have ... become convinced that when we define ourselves by our wounds, we burden and lose our physical and spiritual energy and open ourselves to the risk of illness.'*. In our 'woundology', we struggle with the emotional wounds embedded in our past. While we may not be aware of the wounding that drives the contraction of the lower chakras as discussed up to this point, we are very aware of the emotional wounds that have hit us, like the proverbial arrow, right in the heart. Relationship wounds stemming from our 'family of origin' as well as other relationship difficulties fit into Myss' account of woundology. However, we can experience emotional wounding from other sources as well, such as those tied to the disappointment of unrealized expectations. While we may only be aware of our wounding to some degree (usually cloaked in situational memories), we know that we have been hurt and the memories play like a broken record. They may indeed play so continually that in our grief, we find it difficult to let go and move on. In the contracted Honeysuckle state, we do not expect any happiness, ever.

*Myss, *Why People don't Heal*, p. 6.

As a remedy, Honeysuckle in some ways works like walnut. Walnut assists us in breaking the ties that we need to break in order to move on. Honeysuckle helps to bring us into the present so that we can take advantage of all that it has to offer us. Then we may move forward as our soul intended. Bach described Honeysuckle as the 'Remedy to remove from the mind the regrets and sorrows of the past, to counteract all influences, all wishes and desires of the past and to bring us back into the present'.

If there is one remedy that represents the Divinity found in each of the remedies, it is 'Star of Bethlehem'. This remedy is *the* remedy of comfort for pains and sorrows, according to Bach.† What better remedy for a constricted heart chakra? Traditionally always given for shock, trauma, and grief, this essence seems to promote a release from the wounds that cause us the deepest of hurts. Physical traumas heal; but inasmuch as we are spirit in body, the wounds that cause us the deepest grief are those rooted within us emotionally. These wounds have a symbiotic relationship to Star of Bethlehem that is divinely healing. On the spiritual level, the flower, Star of Bethlehem presents a balanced image of six perfect petals of white, evoking the image of the spiritually-significant six-pointed star, the perfectly counterbalanced triangles, the phrase 'as above, so below' and the culmination of the colours in the spectrum. As a practitioner, I have heard this remedy referred to as the 'ultimate healer of all wounds' and 'the Divine Mother essence'. In other words, it is truly a remedy for a heart in distress.

On our mystic path, it is paramount to keep in mind that

*Chancellor, p. 111. †Chancellor, p. 179.

the will to heal *is* the gateway to our soul's fire. It lies within our spiritual heart. An additional key to this gateway is our ability to embrace and practise the act of forgiveness; forgiveness for ourselves and for others. To find that forgiveness within us requires surrendering the self-imposed guilt and shame that are attached to the contracted issues of the root, sacral and solar plexus chakras. Until we are able to give ourselves permission to take a different path than our family or tribe, to make our own choices and stand in our power within our external environment, we cannot extend forgiveness to others. When we have given ourselves these permissions, then we are better able to forgive others who have hurt us in some way. Moreover, we are burning the karmic debt that is necessary in order to move forward on our mystical path. In his book, *A Path with Heart,* psychologist Jack Kornfield identifies forgiveness as:

> *one of the greatest gifts of the spiritual life. It enables us to be released from the sorrows of the past.... Forgiveness does not in any way justify or condone harmful actions.... Forgiveness is simply an act of the heart, and an acknowledgement that, no matter how strongly you may condemn and have suffered from the evil deeds of another, you will not put another human being out of your heart.*

Then, and only then, will we be able to ask the question, 'did I love enough, *unconditionally',* and get a response that reverberates throughout our deepest levels of awareness.

*Kornfield, pp. 284–5.

CHAPTER THIRTEEN

SPEAK LOUDLY, THOUGH YOUR KNEES QUAKE: THE FIFTH CHAKRA

Agrimony, Cerato, Larch, Chestnut Bud—Wisdom

'How does one become a butterfly?' she asked.
'You must want to fly so much that you are willing to give up
being a caterpillar.'
TRINA PAULUS, *Hope for the Flowers*

SOUND, both spoken and heard, is the energetic element of the fifth centre, our throat. If we review the emotional patterns held within each chakra explored up to this point, we find that within each of them rests aspects of choice. In our first chakra centre, the root, we are faced with the issue of who will make choices for us? Will it be our tribe or ourselves who will determine the direction our path takes? In the sacral and solar plexus centres, we find that our choices affect our empowerment or disempowerment creatively; they shape our personal relationships, our self-esteem and our ability to function in our external environment. Finally coming to this point on our mystical path, we find that the ramifications of the choices we have made in the other centres culminate in our heart centre, affecting our spiritual health.

This assessment now brings us to our fifth chakra, the throat centre. With this centre, we find ourselves at a new frontier, the chakras that are related to our 'spiritual awakening'. We are now embarking into the territory of what the ancients and spiritual teachings identify as the realm of ether or space. With this centre, our relationship to the external earthly realm and the divine within us is established through 'sound'. The question before us is *what is the disposition of this relationship?*

We have learned that we must be faithful in our commitment to do our own emotional work in our lower centres. And, if we have done the work required for our spiritual progress, we have the opportunity to benefit from our labours in the throat centre. The throat centre represents our ability to hear our intuitive wisdom and to speak it. In other words, in its highest expression, the fifth chakra is the centre from which we Speak Our Truth.

> *The unfoldment of the throat chakra will lead the soul to a wider and deeper understanding of the eternal, unchanging truths of life. It is linked with the sense of hearing, both on the physical and spiritual plane, and with the vocal cords and the production of sound.'*

Nevertheless, emotionally and spiritually hearing our wisdom and then speaking it is a formidable challenge when our first four chakras are in contracted states.

If we have not been able to shift the emotional patterns of the root, sacral, solar plexus and the heart chakra into expansion, then the fifth chakra will remain contracted in all aspects as well. Thus, the issue of *speaking our truth* can be fraught with difficulties, as it may be easier for us to speak

*Hodgson, *Stars and Chakras*, p. 138.

our truth than to follow through with what we have said. An authentic journey requires fundamental commitment and action; not simply thinking and talking. For some, when they actually have 'spoken up', their authentic work is embedded in this very action. However, in private practice both myself and other practitioners have all worked with clients who find it very easy to speak up (or out) but have not done the internal work that is required; in other words, their words 'ring hollow' and they are simply giving lip-service to what they are saying. In practice it comes across as verbalizing the current spiritual 'buzz'—or what they think others want to hear—when in actuality, they are unauthentic in their process.

Emotional contraction in the throat chakra prevents us from asking for what we need and thus we are unable to 'speak up.' But how can we 'speak up' if we have been disempowered in the other centres, unable to make choices for ourselves? Furthermore, this contraction prevents us from hearing our intuitive wisdom clearly. Therefore, we can't trust it and are unable to verbalize it. Being unable to speak our truth is only one manifestation of contraction in this centre. Again, sound is the operative characteristic of this chakra and verbalization always carries with it an important responsibility. We choose words to express ourselves and our words transmit powerful vibrations through the ethers. When the throat centre is contracted, our words can emit toxic vibrations to those around us and these vibrations reverberate back to us, creating yet more toxicity within us.

Thus, in this centre, we find that the issue of choice remains within us and has to do with how we communicate our intent, desire, self-direction; our will. If we have done our work in our lower centres, our throat centre will be ready to enter into a state of expansion. This state enables us to hear our intuitive wisdom and speak our own *high truth*. In doing so, we verbalize the intentions of our soul, intentions that represent the balance of our feminine and masculine energies which have been protected in our heart centre.

When we offer words with humble intent, with no expectations, we offer unconditional love in the name of universal connection and service. This does not mean that everyone will accept what we have to say. Additionally, the reality is that the authenticity of unconditional love is not determined by acceptance of our words. It is important to keep in mind that on our journey we are not all reading from the same map; we are not meant to. The understanding of this principle was one that was very clear for Edward Bach and is a concept repeatedly interwoven throughout his writing:

> *We must not expect others to do what we want, their ideas are the right ideas for them, and though their pathway may lead in a different direction from ours, the goal at the end of the journey is the same for us all. We do find that it is when we want others to 'fall in' with our wishes that we fall out with them.'*[*]

From the physical perspective, a contracted throat chakra can manifest as problems in regions of the throat, teeth, mouth, hypothalamus and the vertebrae of the neck. Caroline Myss also identifies addictions as being an indication of fifth-chakra difficulties.[†]

There are a number of remedies that can be considered

*Barnard, *Collected Writings*, p. 102. †Myss, *Anatomy*, p. 98.

when trying to expand a contracted fifth chakra, and each addresses distinctly different emotional issues. In Chapter Six, we learned that Bach identified Agrimony and Cerato as soul-type remedies. But these remedies also are indicated or useful when an individual manifests the contracted emotions of either the temporary mood-state or personality-type of these remedies. In the contracted states, individuals manifesting the Agrimony mood or personality-type hide their true feelings and thus live in intense internal turmoil. In these contracted states, they are not comfortable with *verbally expressing* feelings of distress. Thus, this helplessness is clearly an indication of a contracted throat centre.

In Chapter Five, we saw how contracted state Agrimony soul-types can turn to addictions, particularly drugs and alcohol, as a means of self-medicating in order to manage their distress. The same is true of the contracted mood-state or contracted personality-type. As a healing tool, the remedy Agrimony assists in providing individuals with the feeling that they are in an emotional place of safety and therefore able to verbally express their needs or their distress in an efficacious manner.

The issues of hearing intuitive wisdom, trusting it and expressing it, lie at the heart of the Cerato soul-type, personality-type and the mood-state. The phrase, 'Know Thyself' was inscribed above the entrance to the Temple of Apollo at Delphi, in the sixth century BC. In terms of the fifth chakra, we could expand this phrase to 'know thyself and speak it.' Such is the very essence of the expanded Cerato. In the contracted Cerato mood-state or personality-type, as is true with a contracted Cerato soul, the intuitive voice is heard only as a faint whisper. There is hesitancy in trusting this voice, and a further inability to verbalize it with confidence. As a result, these individuals spend their time doubting every choice they make. This behaviour increasingly promotes their powerlessness internally and certainly, externally in the eyes of all with whom they interact.

Cerato as a remedy promotes the courage needed for effective external expression of inner knowing, of authentic judgment and intuition. The positive energy of the remedy shifts the individuals' internal perspective of themselves, thus amplifying the voice of their intuition and inner knowing. In this space, the individual holds the power of speaking their high truth.

The personality-type and mood-state of *Larch* was discussed in Chapter Eleven. Having to do with issues of self-esteem (a third-chakra issue), this remedy can also be considered as a healing tool for a contracted throat chakra. If we do not possess self-esteem, this dysfunction will be verbalized through a smokescreen of toxic words. This screen only serves to damage others and ourselves. In order to express our desires and needs, self-esteem is essential. Thus, Larch is the remedy to call upon to assist us in this process.

In her book, *The Stars and The Chakras*, the author Joan Hodgson states:

> *The unfoldment of the throat chakra will lead the soul to a wider and deeper understanding of the eternal unchanging truths of life . . . as the throat centre becomes active, the soul begins to feel a longing to communicate—to sound its own individual note in the grand harmony of the universe . . . [but with this] there can be a danger of mental pride and arrogance, barring the path to true spiritual union with the Divine which the soul seeks.*

Here Hodgson cautions us not to let mental pride and arrogance interfere with our ability to make wise choices. When the fifth chakra is contracted, mental pride, arrogance, or a sense of entitlement prevent us from making choices with clear discernment or judgment. In its effort to teach us the importance of discernment in exercising our 'will', our soul provides us with repetitive opportunities through which we can test our progress. Some of the most visible illustrations of these 'soul-opportunities' arise in toxic relationships or life-situations based on unrealistic expectations. Thus, we gauge our progress in learning the soulful skills of sound judgment and clear discernment by our ability to recognize these patterns and reject them.

Recalling that the fifth chakra is about sound, if we continue to ignore our soul's messages through denial and resistance, we can hardly expect to speak with clarity. As a result, we will have to rework this lesson until we 'get it'; and 'getting it' is imperative to discovering our soul's fire. The remedy, *Chestnut Bud* reflects both a mood-state and a personality-type. Recalling that Bach identified the remedies in three categories: soul-type, personality-type and mood-state, we are reminded that all twelve soul-remedies can function as the other two, but he did not consider the balance of the remedies as soul-type remedies. To clarify further, a personality-type remedy represents the chronic emotional state that one's personality presents (which can vacillate between states of expansion and contraction), while the mood state is temporary. Recalling that Bach believed that the personality-type remedies and the mood-state remedies were the ones to consider when addressing illness, we are reminded that these remedies and the emotions they represent are very much about our reactions to our environment.

Chestnut Bud is the remedy Bach chose as the one to help us recognize our repetitive patterns of behaviour, the ones that prevent us from developing clear discernment. By expanding our internal vision, Chestnut Bud has the ability to move us from a contracted state of detrimental repetitiveness into an expanded state that can give us the understanding of the consequences of our actions. However, as with all of the remedies, be they a soul-type, mood-state or personality-type remedy, there *must* be a willingness on the part of the individual to participate in their process. Spiritual teachings remind us that:

> *The difficult part is for a soul to live, day by day, in a dark world absorbing the lessons which the outer life is intended to teach.... Humanity actually spends its time running away from itself, seeking dissipation and oblivion.... [Again, the] essential lesson ... that life has to teach humanity is to face itself.**

As Hodgson implies, when we develop aspects of discernment through these lessons, such as sound judgment, sensitivity, and insight into the choices we make, our fifth chakra expands and we move further along our mystic path toward the acquisition of *Wisdom.*

*White Eagle, *The Light Bringer,* pp. 82–4.

CHAPTER FOURTEEN

IT'S NOT IN YOUR HEAD—
LIGHT-BULB MOMENTS: THE SIXTH
CHAKRA

Cherry Plum and Aspen—Certainty

*'Use your imagination not to scare you to
death, but to inspire you to life'*
ANONYMOUS

VISION, imagination, inspiration, and awareness of our high truth are all channels our soul uses to inform us that we are making progress along our mystical path. The information we receive through these routes comes in 'light-bulb moments' that give us glimpses of our soul-path. Moreover, it is through the centre of the sixth chakra that we 're-ceive divine light.' As a mystic and psychic, Edward Bach became especially sensitive and receptive to such moments during the last two years of his life, particularly with his discovery of the final nineteen remedies. But as early as 1931, when Bach wrote *Heal Thyself,* it can be seen that he was aware of our potential sensitivity to the Divine and our intuition as he refers to such sensitivity as 'flashes of knowledge and guidance [that are] given to us.'*

*Barnard, *Collected Writings*, p. 147.

Making our way upwards through the upper triangle of our chakra symbology, we find that this centre (located above and between our physical eyes) is identified in Eastern philosophy as the 'third eye'. It is in this centre that we have potential access to an innate understanding of the *unknowable*. Successful transition into this 'place' however, requires that we have first transformed the emotional patterns of the first five centres with authenticity; otherwise, we will continue to intellectualize our light-bulb moments and dismiss those that we cannot explain through reductionistic or mechanistic philosophy. As we were reminded at the beginning of Chapter Twelve, the ancient Egyptians believed that successful passage into the underworld was determined by an appraisal of an individual's heart centre against the feather of Maat, the goddess of truth, law, and universal order. Interestingly, we find that other spiritual traditions teach similar concepts although they are expressed differently:

> *Always remember that although words have their place, and are useful to open the door, you cannot advance into the Temple of Initiation on words alone! The passwords on the spiritual plane are not spoken words only. Passwords are sounded in the heart, and you cannot advance ... without sounding the password of the heart centre ... which is love.... You cannot have the power without being love.* *

Thus, transformation of the emotional patterns in the heart centre is particularly important to our progress, for *living* universal brotherhood/sisterhood is grounded in the heart. We need to remember that the power of words and sound, our words grounded in the throat chakra, do not

*White Eagle, *The Light Bringer*, pp. 82–4.

guarantee us an automatic entrée into the place where we receive the 'flashes of knowledge and guidance' to which Bach refers. In order to 'receive' such knowledge, it is essential to remember that the success of our emotional excavations will be deliberated within the heart whether we have lived past lives in ancient Egypt or are simply modern-day travellers. If we have been authentic in the emotional excavation of the lower chakras, and that of the throat, the positive energy of our worldly will in these centres facilitates our heart chakra to open and expand. In an ongoing flow, and as described, this expansion rebounds throughout the other centres in support of their expansion. When our heart centre is open, it becomes a potent sacred space where fusion between the expanded emotional patterns of the lower chakras can take place, with expansion of the sixth centre.

The vibrant emotional and spiritual energy of this centre honours both our conscious and unconscious wisdom. Thus, the language of the sixth centre's wisdom is one that we *feel* through the heart and *verbalize* through our throat chakra. Furthermore, in this state, we become open to light-bulb moments of *vision, imagination, and inspiration, as we become aware of our high truth.*

The sixth chakra centre is also connected to the power of the rational mind. When contracted, the mind emerges as the grasping, hungry ghost, greedy in its desire to dominate to our own detriment. In Bach's view, greed itself fostered a desire for power, manifesting in issues of control. Bach saw greed as the emotion denying the recognition that every soul has the right to freedom and individuality.* It is also

*Barnard, *Collected Writings*, p. 132.

interesting that he identified 'pride' as representing not only arrogance but also rigidity of the mind. Thus, we find that domination by our mind or intellect is not supportive of our mystical path toward soul-awareness. Our intellectual mind does not understand the concept of universal connection, even though this is the greatest lesson that we need to learn as we make our way into the Aquarian Age. Thus, when our intellect dominates, our intuitive wisdom is shut down. Whether we are aware of it or not, we have become prisoners of ourselves and dangerously stuck in our process. In this state, we cannot 'see'; we are blinded to our inner vision and knowing, and it is impossible for us to hear the voice of our intuition.

When we engage in the emotional work necessary to expand the lower chakra centres, various forms of therapy can all be excellent tools (see Chapter One). In addition, the various remedies suggested to this point are all useful in doing our inner work. Beyond the remedies, there are other tools available to us for expanding the upper chakra centres. These are in a different category from the ones used in expanding the lower centres. One of the most powerful is the practice of contemplative prayer and/or meditation. There are excellent resources available though which one might learn methods of meditation including books, tapes and classes. Regardless of the paradigm one chooses, the object of meditative practice is to develop the skill of objective and silent introspection. Bach himself wrote on this subject, remarking:

The perfect method of learning [to obtain a faithful picture of ourselves] is by calm thought and meditation, and by bringing ourselves to such an atmosphere of peace that our Souls are able to speak to us through our conscience and intuition, and to guide us....

While certain remedies are invaluable in assisting us in our quest, it is interesting that Bach is telling us, in so many words, that peaceful silence of contemplative prayer or meditation is *the* key to being able to hear our intuitive guidance; it is not a mental exercise, but one of the heart. This is a message that is given to us by spiritual teachings as well:

When you are distracted by material things, keep very calm, keep very still.... Touch the silence and the power of the spirit will flow into you and disperse all your fears.... 'Nothing is so important as God'. There are many very clever people with great intellectual development, but despite all their knowledge, they are unable to penetrate the higher ethers or touch this profound spiritual silence; and indeed, until you have developed the required spiritual qualities, you will never penetrate these finer ethers.†

Unfortunately, for some, their sacred shopping has derailed them and, as we have already seen, their desire to be 'spiritual' becomes so intense that they make their quest an intellectual one, rather than a spiritual one. We cannot attain expansion of the sixth chakra and our ability to 'receive' through a frenzy of reading books, quoting biblical passages or proselytizing. Silence and authentic introspection are two of the major keys to the expansion of this chakra. Service in the name of unconditional love rather than ego, is yet another powerful key.

The emotional patterns of a contracted sixth chakra can manifest in a variety of dysfunctional and abusive behaviours such as rage, attempts to control others and dictatorial domination. All of these behaviours have been discussed

*Barnard, *Collected Writings*, p. 147. †*The Light Bringer*, p. 39.

in relation to contraction of the other chakras. However, when the sixth centre is in a state of contraction, we can also become what psychologists refer to as delusional. Among the characteristics of this emotional state are delusions of grandeur. In other words, the individual can develop an inflated sense of worth, power, knowledge, or believe that they have a special relationship with a deity or famous person.*

When this happens, they can take on the mantle of a self-professed guru, which not only invites further derailment from their soul's intended mystical path, but derails those whom they beguile as well. We build up access to our soul fire by doing our emotional work with the help of the remedies and introspective meditation. It is important to remember however, that in working toward this access, we must understand that by calling upon the remedies and contemplative meditation, the onus of work still lies with our *active* participation in our process. Solely relying on the remedies to do our work will not reap the results we are after, any more than sitting in contemplative meditation as a phlegmatic observer will bring us enlightenment. While there are many authentic mentors who have travelled their path before us, they are in essence no different from those of us who are 'learning the ropes'. For anyone, success in their process requires that they work through the emotional patterns lodged in their chakras in an orderly fashion.

I tell my clients, 'the minute you hear grandiosity, experience abusive behaviour, language or any other suggestion that a mentor is more interested in you meeting their needs

*Desk Reference to the Diagnostic Criteria from DSM-IV, 1994 edn., p.154.

than the mentor supporting your growth, run the other way. Be especially alert to any needs for adoration on the part of your spiritual advisor or mentor.' This type of need is not supportive of chakra expansion or health.

In addition to its links with our mental capacity, the sixth chakra is physically associated with our brain and central nervous system. When this centre is out of balance, we can experience neurological difficulties, seizures and/or learning disorders. From the spiritual perspective, these manifestations are giving us clues that a spiritual war is raging within us. On one hand the mind, fearful that it will lose its place of importance, is battling for its survival. On the other, our soul is trying to steer us into a place of awareness where we can access our highest truth and *know* what our job is for this lifetime.

From a remedy perspective, these manifestations, emotional and physical, represent the classic struggle between soul and personality agendas. In Chapter Nine, the remedy *Cherry Plum* was introduced as a choice for a contracted first chakra. However, in the case of a contracted sixth centre, when the mind is in its struggle for dominance over the soul, we can also consider this remedy. Cherry Plum was the remedy Bach described for the mind being overworked and unable to take 'strain'. An important consideration of Cherry Plum is its ability to promote internal resolution between mind and soul and thus foster a sense of peace.

Up to this point, the discussion regarding 'contracted emotional chakra patterns' has been one intended to portray an image of centres that are 'closed' like the shutter in a camera just before the picture is snapped. However, the sixth centre presents us with an inconsistency in our imagery. On one hand, when the sixth chakra expands as in the sense of demonstrating balanced emotional patterns, we have an opportunity to access vision, imagination and our high truth. Nevertheless, in this opportunity, we must bear in mind that this is also the centre that fosters our psychic abilities; and in this, there is an inherent danger in expansion, as in being *too open.*

Expanded in an unbalanced way, the sixth centre makes us susceptible and open to 'psychic attack' or 'psychic possession'. In this sense, although the sixth centre is expanded, it is actually out of balance and therefore in a state of contraction. Thus, the individual experiences a type of fear that is so irrational they are afraid to verbalize it to others and lack the language to do so. Their intuition or 'sixth sense' is so skewed that the imagination, rather than being creative and balanced, reels out of control in unrealistic fantasies that are emotionally destructive. In this state, the mind conjures up scenarios, events, and anticipations at a frenetic pace. The results are states of heightened anxiety and/or an intense fear of radical things happening around every corner. It is important to note that these emotions have no tangible basis. A very patent and widespread example of this state was a way of being for most Americans in the days and months following September 11, 2001.

Barnard reminds us that when Bach discovered the final nineteen remedies, he left us with no evidence in his writings as to what specific circumstances initiated this final chapter of his work. The only clues we have are from Nora Weeks. As I pointed out in earlier chapters, she tells us that

Bach experienced specific emotional states of distress just before discovering the remedy that balanced out each particular state of his distress. No doubt, Bach's psychic capabilities were finely tuned to a very high frequency at this point in his life (1935). Thus, it is reasonable to assume that he was susceptible to the implications of a sixth centre that had become too exposed to disquieting influences of a psychic nature. Being open to the etheric plane involves risk for anyone, and this was no less true for Bach. Therefore, we can reasonably assume that this was his experience leading to his discovery of the remedy *Aspen*.

Bach described the contracted Aspen state as experiencing 'an unknown mental fear that comes over you like a cloud, bringing fear, terror, anxiety and even panic without the least reason. These fears are often accompanied with trembling and sweating from the object of fear of something unknown.' Conversely, according to Bach, the positive attributes of the Aspen remedy promote 'fearlessness because of the knowledge that the universal power of love stands behind all. Once we come to that realization, we are beyond pain and suffering, beyond care or worry or fear; we are beyond everything except the joy of life, the joy of death, and the joy of our immortality.... We can walk [our] path through any danger, through any difficulty unafraid.*

Thus, as we strive to obtain a 'faithful picture of ourselves', as Bach called it, we must consciously be aware that *balance* is of the utmost importance in this particular centre. But when we achieve this balance, spiritual teachings tell us that there are marvellous rewards. Open to vision, inspiration,

*Chancellor, p. 43.

imagination, our high truth, and a 'different way of know-ing', we are reminded once again that all great work is done quietly and with *certainty.*

> *When the soul has acquired all the lessons necessary, when it has attained a degree of completeness, it puts forth a more complete presentation of itself. Then you are able to see and recognize a master, an adept, an initiate.*

*White Eagle, *Treasures of the Master Within*, pp.113–14.

CHAPTER FIFTEEN

ILLUMINATION: THE SEVENTH CHAKRA

Sweet Chestnut, Star of Bethlehem—Faith

'Come to the edge', he said. They said, 'we are afraid'.
'Come to edge', he said. They came.
He pushed them ... and they flew'

GUILLAUME APOLLINAIRE

IN THE NATIVE American tradition, young men, and sometimes women (depending on the tribe) undergo a spiritual ritual known as a 'vision quest'. When successful, this ritual of initiation brings the initiate to a place of temporal balance and spiritual adulthood. Though the specifics vary, typically the process includes rituals of purification followed by an intense journey of solitary introspection into the etheric realms. Aided by the individual's spirit guide or animal, this 'journey' provides 'a focus and sense of purpose, personal strength, and power.' In the Shamanic tradition, briefly discussed in Chapter Ten, vision quests also are undertaken in cases of individual problematic circumstances or issues that are affecting the tribe as a whole.

*Harper's Encyclopedia of Mystical and Paranormal Experience, p. 634.

The ritual of a sacred journey into the etheric realms is not exclusive to the Native Americans but is part of every culture and tradition under various labels. For example, in the Christian tradition, one could identify Christ's forty days and forty nights in the desert as his personal 'vision quest'. Within this framework, the upward journey we make through the emotional patterns of our chakras can be considered our personal vision quest in search of our soul's fire. The culmination of this journey is the apex of the upper triangle in our chakra symbology. It is our seventh chakra centre, that of *illumination*. When this centre (located at the crown of the head) is in a state of expansion, we are open to the integration of unconditional surrender to the wisdom of, and faith in, the Divine in every cell within our physical body and every vibration of our etheric bodies.

This is illumination, and it is the Golden Apple sought by the spiritual seeker. It is at the heart of our ultimate connection to all that is Divine within and without us. Thus so 'enlightened', we come to recognize our high truth, our soul fire. *Now* we have the opportunity to embrace this fire and, in doing so, radiate light to others. However, in our attempts to reach this point of completion, we still have to face some difficulties.

For some, impatience develops with the pace of their progress. As a result, they are tempted to evade some (but not necessarily all) of the emotional work needed for discovery of their truth and soul fire. This temptation results in something like a short circuit, wherein through inappropriate practices the individual forces the *kundalini*, the divine fire (or cosmic fire, as it is sometimes called), to rise prema-

turely up through the other chakras. In eastern philosophy, the symbol of this cosmic fire or energy is a coiled ser-
pent lying dormant within the root chakra, which in turn
is located at the base of the spinal column. Spiritual teachings inform us that the kundalini *power* is centred in the heart
and that through gentle meditation, the proper spiritual
awakening that calls for the arousal of this latent energy
can be achieved in an orderly ascension up through the
chakras beginning with the root. When individuals become
impatient and attempt to bypass the orderly work needed
for this process, serious physical difficulties can result.

According to Myss, such imbalances include those within
the central nervous system, the skeletal system, and mus-
cular system of our body, These are, then, red flags for a
seventh chakra whose state is precarious. These imbalances
can manifest in energetic disorders, mystical depression, sen-
sitivities [to the environment] and chronic exhaustion that
is not linked to a physical disorder*

Typically, such disorders are subject to an array of bio-
logically-based diagnoses by those trained in the western
medical tradition. However, in these situations, the difficulty
arises in that the course of treatments recommended often
does not solve the problem. It is not that the methods of
western medicine are substandard, but simply that until very
recently, most western-trained physicians have not been
educated in treating such imbalances from a mind/body/
spiritual perspective; something eastern philosophy and
medicine has considered imperative for thousands of years.
Once again, in this issue of how to treat illness and disease,

*Myss, *Anatomy*, p. 101.

we find that Bach was a visionary in his approach to illness. A saying of his well-known within Bach circles is, 'treat the person, not the disease'. Here he was directly referring to our emotions as the foundation of illness.*

Thus, we find despite some progress our mystical path we still may have some remaining demons and dragons to slay. Therefore, acquiring the Golden Apple of Union with the Divine does not appear to be imminent. Typically, these dragons are the ones that continue to lurk in the comfy lairs of our lower centres. In other words, we have not yet banished them and we still have work to do. Imbalances in the seventh centre can create disillusionment and disconnection throwing us into what St John of the Cross called *the Dark Night of the Soul.* Quite simply, we *believe* that we are in a state of spiritual abandonment. The key here is that we still have not emotionally grasped the concept of *faith in unconditional surrender to the Divine.* The classic description of the constrictive *Sweet Chestnut* state *is* 'dark night of the soul'. Those in the throes of this constrictive state experience unbearable anguish and the perception of assured annihilation. This is a most desperate emotional state for anyone. The abyss which appears to those in this state can create emotional, physical, or spiritual paralysis, and it is not uncommon for an individual to experience all three simultaneously because this chakra centre is either totally contracted or intensely out of balance.

Bach identified the Sweet Chestnut remedy as the one for 'that terrible, that appalling mental despair when it seems

---

*It should be noted that Bach made exceptions to this approach in the cases of catastrophic circumstances such as accidents.

the very soul itself is suffering destruction. [It is] the hopeless despair of those who feel they have reached the limit of their endurance.'

Clearly, Bach must have experienced this state to describe it so. Furthermore, he goes on to say that the positive action of this remedy enables those, despite their anguish, to reach out to the Divine. To this end he said, '...the cry for help is heard and it is the moment when miracles are done.'*

When we find ourselves surrounded by the darkness of our abyss, Sweet Chestnut is the remedy that creates the light we need in order to for us to see through this darkness. Barnard refers to the Sweet Chestnut remedy as the one that is able to 'pull consciousness up from the darkness of [the] underworld.'

In addition to Sweet Chestnut, it is useful to remind ourselves of the remedy that Bach referred to as the 'comforter of pains and sorrows'; Star of Bethlehem. While the specifics of this remedy have been covered in Chapter Twelve, it is interesting to contemplate the image of the flower, Star of Bethlehem, and all of the flowers that Bach chose for healing, within the concept of spiritual teachings:

There is nothing haphazard in creation, all is perfection—perfect rhythm, perfect form, exactness in every detail.... Take a tiny star like flower, and place it under a microscope, and you will see it as a jewel, you will see all the colours of the rainbow reflected in its petals, and if you are attuned to the harmonies of the spheres of light, you will hear them sounding from the beauty of that little flower.... Look for beauty in your everyday life. Do not take things for granted. Look for the exquisite beauty in flowers, in the sunlight, in the dewdrop.†

*Chancellor, p. 186. †White Eagle, *Spiritual Unfoldment 2*, p. 100.

Thus, in order to realize illumination rather than illusion, our seventh centre must be in brilliant and harmonious expansion with our other centres. For this to happen, it is imperative that we have trust and unconditional *faith* that there is a Divine Plan for each of us, expressly orchestrated to inspire transformation that balances us physically, emotionally, and most importantly, spiritually.

CHAPTER SIXTEEN

KEEPING ON KEEPING ON

*The spiritual journey is one of continually
falling on your face, getting up, brushing yourself off, looking
sheepishly at God, and taking another step.*

AUROBINDO

THE CENTRAL theme for humanity in the Aquarian age is internal harmony with our Divine Self and the external harmony of universal connection. While our soul holds this wisdom, some of us—most of us—have disconnected from this wisdom in our frenzy to speed toward and through the wonders of technology. As a mystic and healer, Edward Bach *knew* that in truth, nature is symbiotic with our soul's agenda. This is something the ancients intuitively knew long before the age of technology. *They knew* that all life-energy is connected. Furthermore, they *knew* that it is the Divinity of nature that enfolds and balances us on all levels in our quest for connection to our soul's fire.

In our process, the flower remedies of Edward Bach move us toward the necessary surrender and faith discussed in Chapter Fifteen. In the most subtle of ways, they help us to step out of that space that imprisons us emotionally. They provide us with a haven of emotional safety by fostering a personal introspection and connection to our perceptions and behaviour. In essence, they say to us, 'this is difficult work, but you are safe in doing it'. Bach maintained that our soul holds the innate wisdom for each of us. However, this wisdom becomes clouded when our chakras and their emotional patterns are in a contracted state. It is as if a curtain of fog drops down over this wisdom and we are unable to 'see' clearly. The remedies lift this fog, shifting our perception to a more realistic state of clarity.

When using the remedies, it is common for people to attribute the positive emotional shifts they experience to a myriad of factors; their family, their job, their therapist, none of which factors involve the remedies. This misperception is a classic illustration of the remedies' profound subtlety. Ironically, it is through this very action that they assist us in reclaiming our place on our mystical path, providing us opportunity and giving us a vision of the intimate relationship we have with the spiritual realm. Furthermore, the remedies help us tap into our reality so that we understand who we are in our quest to discover and manifest our soul's fire. For Bach, the understanding of our spiritual reality was his *high truth*.

Within the realms of cosmic law, there is the concept of soul-age, similar to the concept of our physical age in the mundane world. As we travel the cycle of birth, death and rebirth, we have many opportunities to learn valuable soul-lessons and as we stumble, get up, dust ourselves off, move on, and sometimes succeed along the way, our soul ages in wisdom. Edward Bach was not only a mystic and healer. He was a *great soul, an old soul*.

Bach's gift to us was one of selflessness. Such a gift is an important quality that is necessary in all of us if we are to achieve the divine mandate of universal connection in brother–sisterhood. While those who worked with him admit that he was not always an easy person to be with, his capacity of compassion for all other human beings was paramount. Most probably, his own consciousness of having a specific job to do in this incarnation, and that nonetheless time was fleeting, was what drove him in his states of impatience and intensity. Although he paid a high price physically, his insatiable passion to find a means of helping others heal their minds and bodies through nature was his mission. For him, finding one's soul-path, discovering what ignites the soul's fire, through purpose and connection, were *the* reasons for being.

We will never know the intimate details of Bach's personal 'flashes of knowledge and guidance' that led him to his discoveries. Regardless of this, the foundation of his work and his words are clearly anchored in spirit. He repeatedly urges us to manifest all that *we are* in spirit. Over and above his work as a physician, this was his reason for being. His own wisdom informs us that our healing and soul-growth depend upon the balance of our emotional energy. For Bach the life-force or positive energy of nature held the keys to healing and soul-growth. It is the 'flash of knowledge' we get as the keys turn that is the divine alchemy of universal connection, brotherhood and unity between all peoples.

For these things, our gratitude to Edward Bach is immeasurable.

The gaining of our freedom, the winning our individuality and independence, will in most cases call for much courage and faith. But in the darkest hours, and when success seems well-nigh impossible, let us ever remember that God's children should never be afraid, that our souls only give us such tasks as we are capable of accomplishing, and that with our own courage and faith in the Divinity within us victory must come to all who continue to strive.

Edward Bach, M.B., B.S., M.R.C.S., L.R.C.P., D.P.H

THE 38 BACH FLOWER REMEDIES

Alphabetical List

Agrimony*

Aspen

Beech

Centaury*

Cerato*

Cherry Plum

Chestnut Bud

Chicory*

Clematis*

Crab Apple

Elm

Gentian*

Gorse

Heather

Holly

Impatiens*

Larch

Mimulus*

Mustard

Oak

Olive

Pine

Red Chestnut

Rock Rose*

Rock Water

Scleranthus*

Star of Bethlehem

Sweet Chestnut

Vervain*

Vine

Walnut

Water Violet*

White Chestnut

Wild Oat

Wild Rose

Willow

Indicates the Twelve Healers and Soul Types

PRACTICAL MATTERS

While there are many flower remedy repertoires available all over the world, it is generally accepted that all of them, even with their variances, are based on Dr Bach's work. Because there are so many, including those provided by cottage-industry enterprises, it is difficult to be familiar with all the available sources. Thus, I can only provide information on those with whom I am personally familiar. In the UK, there are two major manufacturers that I am aware of. Both repertoires offer thirty-eight remedies replicated from the varieties of the thirty-seven flowers and rock water originally chosen by Dr Bach. The *Bach Flower Remedies* through A. Nelson, Ltd (in collaboration with The Dr Bach Centre, Oxfordshire) are available at a great many chemists and health stores. Additionally, the remedies offered by Julian Barnard's *Healing Herbs, Ltd.* (Herefordshire) are also readily obtainable through healthcare practitioners, natural health shops and some chemists.

As a rule, flower remedies in the United States are sold as flower 'essences' in order to comply with the US Federal Drug and Food Administration labelling requirements, lest there be any confusion over terms. As with the availability in the UK, flower essences in the US are available in natural food stores and through large, national sources such as the Whole Foods Markets and Wild Oats Markets.

Major repertoires available in the US that are based on Dr Bach's original thirty-eight include the Bach Flower Essences (NelsonBach, USA, Wilmington, Massachusetts) and the essences from the Flower Essence Society (FES) located in Culver City, California. The FES repertoire offers a broad range of remedies made from Native North

American Flowers and very importantly, this repertoire also includes Julian Barnard's thirty-eight *Healing Herbs,* mentioned above. Additional repertoires worth noting of which I am personally familiar are the Desert Alchemy group (Tucson, Az), made from desert flowers, and the Perelandra group (Warrenton, Va). The Perelandra repertoire is very extensive in its offerings, philosophy, and worth investigating. There are several other repertoires available in the US as well as those from other countries through the internet, particularly those in South America, Japan and Australia.

Fair Warning: when selecting remedies, it is always wise to research the source, background and philosophy of those who are providing them. Over the years I have come across repertoires whose philosophy circumvents the need for doing the very earthly emotional work, in exchange for spiritual illumination. Such claims and marketing are not only 'airy fairy', but charlatanistic in intent and definitely not in the spirit of Dr Bach's philosophy.

In creating a system of healing, Dr Bach's objective was to find a system that would be simple to incorporate into one's everyday lifestyle. The following information is intended to provide very general guidelines.

GENERAL GUIDELINES FOR THE BACH REMEDIES

In addressing temporary mood-states or negative personality-characteristics, selection of the appropriate remedies is made according to 'key indicators'. Keeping in mind that there are over two hundred million possible combinations of the thirty-eight, more extensive guidance (in addition to those discussed in Chapters Nine to Fifteen) may be found in the available resources listed under 'Further Reading', below.

¶ Although homeopathic in nature, the remedies are not made from any plants or parts of plants that are poisonous

¶ They can be used at any time of day without concern of potency negation due to food or drink of any type.

¶ In the case of the individual thirty-eight remedies, a single dosage is two drops, with a frequency of four times per day, or more if the individual feels the need. These can be taken directly in the tongue or in a glass of spring water or juice, for sipping.

¶ The Bach remedies offered by both NelsonBach Ltd., and Healing Herbs, Ltd. are preserved in brandy. For those who are alcohol-sensitive or prefer not to ingest alcohol, the remedies may be applied to the pulse points (in the same dosage as if taken under the tongue). They can also be used in the bath (five to six drops), massage oils (five to six drops) or in a spray bottle to mist a room (five to six drops), for example.

¶ The remedies can also be added to your watering can (for plants, ten drops per gallon) or water bowls for animals (two drops for small animals, ten per gallon for larger animals), for example. For small animals, they can also be applied to the paws, nose or placed in the mouth.

PERSONAL FORMULA

Dr Bach recognized that often there was a call for more than one remedy at a time and that such combination might be needed over an extended period of time. Such combinations are especially called for when an individual is struggling with deeper emotional issues than those of a temporary nature, such as grief. In practice, the number of essences in a 'personal formula' is traditionally limited from five to seven, depending on the manufacturer. Such a formula is made by filling a sterilized 30ml dropper bottle with spring water. To this, 2 drops of each of the chosen remedies is added. Additional brandy or other drinking alcohol may be added to top off the formula with the purpose of stabilizing the water. This is not necessary, but is useful in warm climates. Dosage is four drops, four times (or more) per day. Such a bottle should last three to four weeks. Dr Bach felt that at least one 'personal formula bottle' should be finished before considering changes to the formula.

RESCUE REMEDY

Before he settled at Mt Vernon, Bach spent the winter of 1933 and the early spring of 1934 in Cromer (Norfolk) where, Weeks reports, he saw patients and 'continued to gain a greater understanding of the properties of the new remedies'.* At some point during this time, Bach made up a combination of Rock Rose, Clematis and Impatiens, which he called the 'Rescue Remedy' to be used in case of emergency, shock, accident, great pain, fear or unconsciousness. She goes on to report that he later added two more remedies to this combination and while we have no information as to specifics, we can speculate that they were Cherry Plum and Star of Bethlehem that complete the combination we know today as Dr Bach's Rescue Remedy. Both remedies are among the final nineteen that he discovered after he moved to Mt Vernon in April of 1934.

Today Dr Bach's formula is known the world over as *the* remedy to call upon in times of mild to extreme stress, trauma or other emergencies. 'Rescue' stories are legendary and as a practitioner, I have heard hundreds, some quite dramatic, and I am never without it. It is available in liquid or spray forms (dosage four drops or two sprays, as needed) and in cream form (for topical palliative uses, with the addition of Crab Apple). These are available under the label, *Rescue Remedy* through A. Nelson's (UK) or Nelson Bach, USA., Ltd. Dr Bach's formula is also found in Julian Barnard's *Healing Herbs* repertoire, in both liquid and cream, under the label, *Five Flower Formula.*

For those interested in the specific healing dynamics found in Dr Bach's 'Rescue' formula, please refer back to Chapter Five (The Twelve Great Remedies) for profiles on Clematis, Impatiens, and Rock Rose. Abbreviated profiles for Cherry Plum may be found in Chapters Nine and Fourteen, Star of Bethlehem in Chapters Twelve and Fifteen, and Crab Apple appears in Chapter Ten.

*Weeks, *Discoveries*, p. 103.

SELECTED FURTHER READING

Dr Bach's own writings are to be found assembled by Julian Barnard in his *Collected Writings*, below, and in the edition of *Original Writings,* edited by Howard and Ramsell, listed below under their own names.

Bach, Edward. *Collected Writings of Edward Bach.* Ed. Julian Barnard. London: Ashgrove Publishing, 1987.

Ballantine, Rudolph. *Radical Healing: Integrating the World's Great Therapeutic Traditions to create a New Transformative Medicine.* New York: Harmony, 1999.

Barnard, Julian. *Bach Flower Remedies: Form & Function.* Hereford: Flower Remedy Programme, 2002.

Dr Philip M. Chancellor's Handbook of the Bach Flower Remedies, Keats Publishing, New Canaan, Ct. 1971

Dossey, Barbara. *Florence Nightingale: Mystic, Visionary, Healer.* New York, Lippincott, Williams & Wilkins, 1999.

Gerber, Richard. *Vibrational Medicine for the Twenty-First Century: The Complete Guide to Energy Healing and Spiritual Transformation.* New York: Eagle Book, Harper Collins, 2000.

Hasnas, Rachelle. *The Essence of Bach Flowers: Traditional and Transpersonal Use and Practice.* Freedom, Ca.: Crossing Press, 1999.

Hay, Louise. *You Can Heal Your Life.* Santa Monica, Ca.: Hay House, 1984.

Hodgson, Joan. *Astrology: The Sacred Science.* Hampshire: The White Eagle Publishing Trust, 1978.

——, *The Stars and the Chakras.* Hampshire: The White Eagle Publishing Trust, 1990.

Howard, Judy, and John Ramsell. *The Original Writings of Edward Bach.* Essex: C.W. Daniel Co., Ltd., 1990.

Kornfield, Jack. *A Path With Heart: A Guide Through the Perils and Promises of Spiritual Life.* New York: Bantam, 1993.

Myss, Caroline. *Anatomy of Spirit.* New York: Harmony Books, 1996.

——, *Why People Don't Heal and How They Can.* New York: Harmony Books, 1997.

Rinpoche, Sogyal. *The Tibetan Book of Living and Dying.* Patrick Gaffney and Andrew Harvey, Eds. San Francisco: HarperCollins, 1993.

Teasdall, Wayne. *The Mystic Heart.* Novato, Ca.: New World Liby., 2001.

Weeks, Nora. *The Medical Discoveries of Edward Bach, Physician: What the Flowers do for the Human Body.* Essex: C. W. Daniel Co., Ltd. , 1973.

White Eagle. *The Light Bringer: The Ray of John and the Age of Intuition.* Hampshire: White Eagle Publishing Trust, 2001.

——, *The Path of the Soul: The Great Initiations.* Hampshire: White Eagle Publishing Trust, 1997.

——, *Treasures of the Master Within.* Hampshire: White Eagle Publishing Trust, 2002.

——, *White Eagle on the Great Spirit*, White Eagle Publishing Trust, 2003

CITATIONS IN TEXT NOT FOUND IN 'FURTHER READING'

Bell, Rudolph M. *Holy Anorexia.* Chicago: Univ. Chicago Press, 1997

Cameron, Julia. *The Artist's Way.* New York: Tarcher, Putnam, 1992.

Harper's Encyclopedia of Mystical & Paranormal Experience. 1991.

Ingerman, Sandra. 'Medicine for the Earth, Medicine for People.' *Alternative Therapies in Medicine and Health* 9:6 (2003) 77-84.

Mack, Gaye. 'Exploring Implications of Treating Eating Disorders with Vibrational Medicine as an Integrative Therapy.' 1999 ,DePaul University., Chicago, Illinois.

Pert, Candace. 'Candace Pert, Ph. D: Neuropeptides, Aids, and the Science of Mind-Body Healing.' *Alternative Therapies in Medicine and Health* 1:3 (1995), pp. 70–6.

White Eagle. *Stella Polaris*, 1952, pp. 18–19, 184.

——, *Spiritual Unfoldment 2.* Hampshire: White Eagle Publishing Trust, 2002.

polair publishing

'the great little publisher for the new age'

THE WORLD IS IN MY GARDEN Chris Maser with Zane Maser
Internationally-acclaimed environmentalist Chris Maser shows how ecological, social, personal and spiritual issues can all be understood through the choices each one of us has to make in our own garden. His wife, Zane, takes us further, into the world of meditation.

September 2003 · ISBN 0-9545389-0-0 · £9.99

YOUR YOGA BODYMAP FOR VITALITY Jenny Beeken
This book has changed the way yoga postures can be taught, because uniquely it works from each area of the body (feet and ankles, sacrum and belly, neck and head, etc.) into a programme of postures. It is particularly suitable for those leading an active life. Sue Peggs' brilliant stop-action photography makes the postures unusually easy to follow.

November 2003 · ISBN 0-9545389-1-9 · £15.99

THE HAMBLIN COURSE IN MYSTICISM
Mark C. W. Sleep brings to light thirty-six rediscovered lessons by Henry Thomas Hamblin and Joel S. Goldsmith, which with commentary and exercises make a complete course in mysticism. You can indeed heal your life through this positive approach.

May 2004 · ISBN 0-9545389-5-1 · £13.99

THE SHAKESPEARE ENIGMA. Peter Dawkins.
Shakespeare himself let slip some words about 'both your poets' which are the first clue in unravelling an extraordinary story that puts the question 'Who wrote Shakespeare?' into a whole new prominence. Peter's holistic approach is itself a huge contribution to enjoyment of what we call 'the Shakespeare plays'.

May 2004 · ISBN 0-9545389-4-3 · £16.99

Forthcoming titles include ROSE ELLIOT'S GLOBAL KITCHEN —a book about ingredients from around the world by Britain's best-known vegetarian cookery writer.

www.polairpublishing.co.uk